Baby Treatment Based on NDT Principles

Lois Bly, M.A., PT

Foreword by Allison Whiteside
Photographs by Ron Medvescek

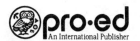

8700 Shoal Creek Boulevard
Austin, Texas 78757-6897
800/897-3202   Fax 800/397-7633
www.proedinc.com

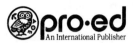

© 1999 by PRO-ED, Inc.
8700 Shoal Creek Boulevard
Austin, Texas 78757-6897
800/897-3202   Fax 800/397-7633
www.proedinc.com

ISBN-13: 978-141640269-5
ISBN-10: 1-41640269-1

Previously published by Therapy Skill Builders, a division of
The Psychological Corporation, under ISBN 0761644504.

Printed in the United States of America

6 7 8 9 10 11 12 13 14 15   27 26 25 24 23 22 21 20 19 18

Dedication

This book is dedicated to Mary Quinton, physiotherapist, and Elsbeth Kong, MD, pediatrician of Bern, Switzerland, the pioneers of "NDT Baby Treatment" as we know it today. These gifted women identified subtle movement problems in babies that, left untreated, would develop into major problems. Not only did they identify these subtle problems, they developed specific treatment and facilitation techniques to minimize and, in many cases, eliminate the problems and thus prevent the numerous compensatory problems that occur in children with cerebral palsy. They have been instrumental in changing the course of cerebral palsy.

Thank you, Dr. Elsbeth Kong and Mary Quinton, for touching the lives of babies and therapists throughout the world!

Acknowledgments

I extend my heartfelt gratitude to everyone who helped make this book a reality.

I would like to thank the following individuals and organizations for the use of their therapy equipment and for helping find the babies:

- Allison Whiteside with Building Blocks—Therapy for Infants and Toddlers
- Marsha Klein and Jill Martindale with Pueblo Pediatric Therapy
- The Van Maren Family
- The Offret Family
- Newborn Intensive Care Program, Tucson Developmental Follow-Up Clinic for Families
- Julie Feldman and her birthing group friends

The babies are the heart of this book and, of course, they captured the hearts of each of us who worked with them and everyone who came to observe. Thank you to all of the babies: Jennifer Arana, Kyle Belson, Erika Cook, Thomas Cordova, Dominic Cozzens, Rachel Dveirin, Michael Forte, Joshua Giordano, Kyra Giordano, Marcos Gonzales, Rachel Gough, Ryan Green, Olivia Habbestad, Guy Lindstrom, Petra Maestas, David Martinez, Matthew McCarthy, Austin Ortiz, RikkiMarie Santa Cruz, Caylor Schuldt, Taylor Seitz, Karissa Sheehey, Reid Sinclair, and Brandon Smalling.

My appreciation also goes to all of the parents and family members who enthusiastically brought their babies to the photography sessions and cheered them on.

Thank you to Allison and Steve Whiteside for welcoming me into their home during the photography sessions.

Thank you to the Medvescek family. Ron and Chris were very supportive and encouraging. Their children Sarah, Nicholas, and Eli were captivated by the babies and, if given the choice, would have stayed home from school to play with each of the babies.

Of course, I could never have completed this book without the rest of the team, Ron Medvescek and Allison Whiteside.

My deepest gratitude goes to Ron Medvescek, whose obvious talent as a photographer is enhanced by his ability to make me feel comfortable. He captured the essence and flow of the movements, even when the babies did not "pose" for the shots. His spirit relaxed and captured the personality of each baby. Everyone should have the opportunity to work with someone like Ron.

My eternal thanks go to Allison Whiteside, without whose support, encouragement, and organization this book might never have been written. She found all of the babies, arranged the schedules, and organized all of the photography sessions. She was my personal chauffeur and make-up artist, the producer and director of the photography sessions, and she kept the "show" running. But most of all, I appreciate her loyal friendship.

My boundless thanks go to the Creator. I never would have had the courage to embark on this project without His encouraging words. "Do not fear, for I am with you; do not be dismayed, for I am your God. I will strengthen you and help you..." (Isaiah 41:10).

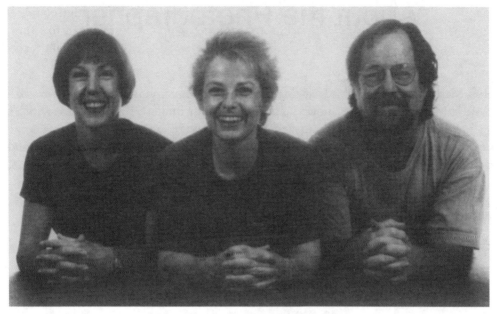

Author Lois Bly (center), Allison Whiteside (left), and photographer Ron Medvescek (right).

About the Author

Lois L. Bly, M.A., PT, received her bachelor of arts, with a major in biology, from Thiel College in Greenville, Pennsylvania, and a certificate of physical therapy from the D. T. Watson School of Physiatrics in Leetsdale, Pennsylvania. She did graduate work in pathokinesiology at New York University, New York, New York, and received her Master of Arts degree in Motor Learning from Teachers College, Columbia University, New York, New York.

Ms. Bly received her initial training in Neuro-Developmental Treatment (NDT) from Dr. and Mrs. Bobath in London, England. She also has attended numerous NDT courses, including the NDT Baby Course with Ms. Mary Quinton and Dr. Elsbeth Kong in Bern, Switzerland. Following the Baby Course, Ms. Bly worked and studied at the Inselspital Bern, Zentrum fur Cerebrale Bewegungsstorungen, Bern, Switzerland. After a 10-week course with Ms. Quinton and Dr. Kong in Seattle, Washington, Ms. Bly became an NDT Coordinator Instructor and was certified to teach 8-week NDTA, Inc., Courses and NDTA Approved Baby Courses.

Ms. Bly is the author of the monograph *The Components of Normal Movement During the First Year of Life* and the book *Motor Skill Acquisition in the First Year* and coauthor with Allison Whiteside of the book *Facilitation Techniques Based on NDT Principles.*

Ms. Bly has worked for many years as a physical therapist, treating babies with developmental disabilities and children with cerebral palsy. Since 1980, she has taught numerous seminars, workshops, NDT basic courses, and advanced Baby Courses throughout the United States, Australia, Brazil, Argentina, and South Africa. Currently she continues to teach, consult, and maintain a very small private practice in Maryland.

About the Photographer

Ron Medvescek received his bachelor of science degree in photojournalism from Ball State University in Muncie, Indiana. He is an award-winning photojournalist with 21 years of experience in newspaper and magazine photography, picture editing, page design, and computer illustration. In addition, he has taught photojournalism and publication design at the University of Arizona. Various magazines and newspapers, such as *Newsweek* and the *Chicago Tribune,* have published some of his work. His photos also appear in Lois Bly's and Allison Whiteside's *Facilitation Techniques Based on NDT Principles.*

Contents

Foreword

Lois Bly is best known within the pediatric therapy community of North America as the foremost expert in the treatment of infants and babies. Lois graciously has acknowledged Mary Quinton, PT, as the founder of baby treatment and as her mentor throughout the years. This publication is a tribute to Mary Quinton and her discoveries in the successful treatment of babies with neuromotor dysfunction. Lois must be commended for putting Mary Quinton's thoughts, ideas, lectures, and facilitation techniques and her own studies of biomechanics, kinesiology, motor learning, and motor control into a well-organized publication.

This publication brings the pediatric therapy community a written guide for clinical, hands-on treatment of babies. Until now, pediatric therapists have had to rely upon co-workers to share their knowledge from NDT courses, or have had to attend a lengthy NDT course, take copious notes to describe the treatment techniques, or be gifted as an artist and draw the techniques. I have been privileged to take two NDT Advanced Baby Courses and each time dreamed of a publication or a manual that would have photographs and a description of each technique. Because there was no such publication, I had to rely upon the written word and considerable practice with a doll before I had the confidence in my skills to treat a baby effectively.

This publication comes at a critical time in the managed care and outcome-based treatment of children with special needs. Due to budget limitations, many therapists are unable to go away for the 8-week Pediatric NDT course followed by the 2- or 3-week Advanced Baby Course. Therefore, therapists can use this publication as a self-study guide for the treatment of babies or as a guide for department education within a hospital, clinic, private practice, or school-based program. This book organizes the treatment techniques around functional goals the baby can attain by problem-solving movement strategies. Treatment goals must reflect that the baby has attained new motor skills for managed care to assess progress and to understand the efficacy of treatment with babies.

I commend Lois for openly sharing her knowledge with the pediatric therapy communities of North America, South America, Europe, and South Africa. The publication of this book is yet another of her efforts to disseminate information that will enhance the lives of children with cerebral palsy and acheive her lifelong dream to see the cure of cerebral palsy.

Thank you, Lois, for your openness to learn and share your knowledge. It is through the open sharing of our knowledge, treatment assumptions, treatment approaches, treatment organization, and critical assessment of functional outcomes that we will find the way to enhance the lives of all children!

Allison Whiteside, PT

Preface

The handling and facilitation involved in baby treatment are among the most precise forms of therapeutic exercise. A therapist's handling can give the baby experiences of typical movements and typical movement sequences that can enhance the baby's development of motor learning skills. The movement experiences you provide can help the baby learn how to solve difficulties in performing motor skills in a variety of ways. Your handling can help the baby learn typical, efficient movements rather than atypical, stereotyped movements.

How you handle and facilitate the baby are very important. Always consider kinesiological issues such as alignment, joint mobility, and muscle activation because the baby's musculoskeletal system is in the process of developing and therefore is very vulnerable to input. Sensory issues are of particular importance in baby treatment because sensory feedback is a major channel of motor learning.

This book provides suggestions on handling babies to improve the quality and repertoire of their movements. Most of the facilitation techniques presented and described in this book, *Baby Treatment Based on NDT Principles,* stem from facilitation techniques created by Mary Quinton. She transformed her visual observations of babies, who were developing typically, and her gifted understanding of movement into creative and gentle ways to help babies with movement disturbances learn how to move.

In many ways, *Baby Treatment Based on NDT Principles* is the basis of *Facilitation Techniques Based on NDT Principles* (1997) that I wrote with Allison Whiteside. The facilitation techniques in both books have evolved from those originally created and taught by Mary Quinton, who was the instructor of my original NDT Baby Course in Bern, Switzerland. At that time I had no idea how Mary Quinton would change and enrich my professional life.

It was in that NDT Baby Course that I first was *exposed* to "baby facilitation techniques." Four months after I took the course, I returned to Bern to work for 2 months, to *learn* how to treat babies. After I returned home, I continued to practice and use the baby techniques. I used them on all of the babies and children with whom I worked. Eventually, I realized that not all of the techniques were appropriate for older children and that those that were appropriate required modification or adaptation to their needs. Subsequently, I separated the techniques into those for babies and those for older children.

In the NDT Baby Course in Bern, and in other courses that I have taken with her, Mary Quinton taught and shared the baby treatment techniques that she had developed. Her teaching was unique in that it was almost entirely experiential. She emphasized how important it was for each of us to experience the movements we would use to treat babies so that we could get the movements into our own body image. I continue to use this method of teaching in my courses. I highly recommend that you also experience the postures and movements of the babies you are treating. The experience will be very enlightening.

In Ms. Quinton's courses, we also used dolls to practice the techniques. By using dolls, we could practice the techniques and develop our coordination and skill without subjecting babies to our clumsy learning process. Of course, treating a doll is much easier than treating a real baby. I continue to use this method of teaching in all of my courses. I highly recommend that you practice each of the techniques with a doll before trying them on a baby. Facilitating a doll also is a good way to demonstrate the techniques to parents and other caregivers.

There were no handouts in Mary Quinton's courses, and none of her genius in treating babies has been published. (However, there is a series of five movies in which Ms. Quinton treats a baby over a 1-year period.) During Ms. Quinton's courses, I tried to write down the techniques so that I would not forget them. My drawings and original descriptions left much to be desired. However, because of my learning experiences with Ms. Quinton, I went back and practiced the postures and movements on myself and on a doll to try to reinforce my "motor memory." I continue to be thankful that Ms. Quinton made me aware of and opened that channel of learning for me.

Unfortunately, most therapists will not have the opportunity to take a course from Mary Quinton. However, I trust that many will continue to learn from her through this book, *Baby Treatment Based on NDT Principles*.

Although the facilitation techniques presented in this book have their origins in the work of Mary Quinton, I have added my own understanding and perspective to the process and art of facilitation. I have added the emphasis on the kinesiological and biomechanical components and the need to address the sensory components of motor learning. I take full responsibility for any unintentional misrepresentation I may make of Ms. Quinton's work. I have worked with and taught the material in this book for many years. I continue to teach "Baby Courses" that vary in length from 1 to 3 weeks.

Baby Treatment Based on NDT Principles is a companion book to my two other books: *Motor Skills Acquisition in the First Year* (1994) and *Facilitation Techniques Based on NDT Principles* (Bly & Whiteside, 1997), written with Allison Whiteside.

Motor Skills Acquisition in the First Year (1994) is a worthy companion in that it describes and illustrates how babies typically move so easily, how they solve motor challenges, and how they practice and develop a variety of motor skills. Babies who have developmental delays, cerebral palsy, and/or other motor dysfunctions have difficulty moving. They have difficulty with solving motor challenges, and they are limited in the variety of their motor skills and often develop and use very stereo-typed movements.

You will find that the outline of this book, as well as many of the descriptions and explanations, are the same as those in *Facilitation Techniques Based on NDT Principles*. We thought that it was important to have two books even though there are many duplications. The content of each book is unique in the type, size, and age of clients being treated. For babies, you must use hand placements, body positions, movements, and body mechanics that are different from those you use with older clients. You also must interact differently with a baby in order to monitor closely and change the baby's state, attention, and physiological status.

Each chapter consists of many facilitation techniques. A stated treatment/movement goal introduces each technique, followed by the baby's position, therapist's position, therapist's hand placement, movement, precautions, component goals, and functional goals. In addition to the detailed directions, many sequential photographs illustrate each facilitation technique.*

Each section describes the component goals for each facilitation technique in detail. Functional goals are more vague because they need to be specific to the motivation and interests of individual babies. I strongly believe that all therapy must be functionally oriented and directed. Therapists must incorporate these functional goals into each treatment session. I do not believe that just providing the components will enable the baby to incorporate them automatically into functional goals.

Photographs and written explanations illustrate and describe each of the techniques in the 12 chapters: Supine, Supine Rolling, Prone on Lap, Prone on Ball, Prone on Floor, Prone on Bolster, Floor Transitions, Sitting on Lap, Sitting on Lap Sequences, Sitting on Ball, Sitting on Bolster, and Standing and Walking.

You must use professional judgment and careful administration in the selection and use of any of the techniques with any baby. Not all of the techniques are appropriate for all babies. If any baby has difficulty with any of the facilitation techniques, you must **never** try to force the baby through the facilitation. Instead, modify or temporarily abandon the facilitation. Do not attempt to use a facilitation technique that would compromise the baby's safety. **The baby's safety and comfort always must be the primary consideration.**

Your safety is also a concern. You need to know your strengths and abilities to handle babies with various degrees of impairments and disabilities. Always use good body mechanics to prevent and avoid personal injury.

The photographer photographed 24 charming babies ranging in age from 4 months to 13 months for this book. Ten of the babies were born prematurely; three of the babies had a diagnosis of Down Syndrome; and two had a diagnosis of developmental delay. We selected the babies to demonstrate the facilitation techniques, not to demonstrate impairments. The goal of the book is to demonstrate specific facilitation techniques, not to treat specific impairments.

All of the babies came from the Tucson, Arizona, area. The parents volunteered to have their babies photographed for a textbook in response to notices placed in the offices of pediatricians and the Tucson Developmental Follow-Up Clinic for Families and word of mouth from friends. We selected Tucson because the homes of my valuable assistant, Allison Whiteside, PT, and photographer Ron Medvescek are in Tucson and I love visiting Arizona.

Conclusion

Facilitation techniques are not synonymous with treatment techniques. Treatment is much more encompassing. You must design treatment to address each baby's specific interests, strengths, and impairments. Facilitation techniques are one—albeit important—facet of treatment. They are a means by which you can help the baby engage in activities that are interesting, while using innate strengths and reducing impairments that limit or prevent such participation. Facilitation techniques enable the baby to experience a variety of movements and add to the baby's repertoire of movements. Although you help the baby through the movements, the experiences can help the baby solve movement challenges more effectively and decrease the chances of, or altogether prevent, the baby's learning stereotyped positions and/or movements. Regardless of which facilitation techniques you use, incorporate them into a functional activity or goal that is meaningful for the baby. Play and exploration of body parts is functional for babies. This will facilitate the baby's use of the movement in real life.

It is my hope and prayer that this book will help you to help many babies discover their unique possibilities.

---

* Some of this material previously appeared in *Facilitation Techniques Based on NDT Principles*, 1997.

Introduction

Principles of Baby Treatment

Treating a baby is both a joy and an awesome responsibility. Babies are fun to work with because they are cute, small, easy to hold and handle, and receptive to treatment.

Treating a baby is an awesome responsibility to accept because you help shape the baby's development by how you structure the therapeutic environment and how you instruct the caregivers. The baby is very vulnerable to handling and to the environment because of the plasticity of the developing systems. All experiences in the extrauterine world are new experiences to the baby.

In the early months of life, all of the sensory systems (visual, tactile, proprioceptive, kinesthetic, vestibular, auditory, and olfactory) impose incredible degrees of sensory stimulation on the baby. The baby must learn how to regulate all of the incoming stimuli in order to be in an optimal state to learn new skills.

Although this regulation usually occurs in the early months of the baby's life, it is important to assess each baby's ability to regulate incoming sensory stimuli regardless of the baby's age. When the baby is content, alert, moves smoothly, and breathes regularly, we assume that the baby's regulatory skills are functioning appropriately. When the baby is stressed or not alert, we must determine the cause of the stress or lack of interest and decrease the stress and potential sources.

Babies who are medically fragile also may have problems with behavioral state regulation and stress management. It is imperative, when working with fragile babies, to become knowledgeable about the baby's medical status, contraindications, precautions, and symptoms of stress. Learn to recognize and manage physiological changes that may arise while you are working with the baby. If you are planning to treat babies who are medically fragile, it is extremely important that you participate in a mentorship or training with an experienced professional preceptor.

State Regulation and Stress Signs

A critical component of treatment of babies is awareness of the baby's stress signs. Stress indicates that the baby is not functioning optimally and therefore will have difficulty learning the movements you are trying to teach. Stress also can be detrimental to the baby's health and well-being. Although crying is an obvious sign of stress, most babies give signals of stress before they actually cry.

Although developed for specific use with neonates, Als' *Synactive Model of Neonatal Behavioral Organization* (1986) is valuable for examining, evaluating, and monitoring all babies during treatment. In this model, the therapist observes the continuous interaction of the baby's three behavioral systems (i.e., autonomic system, motor system, and state system) in relation to the baby's interaction with the environment. Als suggests that the baby communicates through these three behavioral systems and refers to this communication as "behavioral language" (Als, 1997, p. 969).

The **autonomic system** is responsible for regulation of respiration, cardiac function/color, and visceral stability. When the baby is stable and organized, these systems function smoothly. When the baby is stressed, there can be changes in this system. Some of the indications of stress are changes in the respiratory pattern, yawning, coughing, hiccuping, color changes such as mottling or cyanosis, temperature changes, trembling, spitting up, bowel movements, tremors, startles, or possibly seizures (Als, 1986, 1996, 1997).

According to synactive theory, when the baby is organized and not stressed, the **motor system** functions easily, with smooth movements and postures. When the baby is stressed, posture and movements may become hypertonic or hypotonic or fluctuate between the two. The hypertonic behaviors include marked extension of the trunk and extremities, scapular retraction with a high-guard position of the arms, finger extension or finger fisting, and facial grimaces. Hypotonic behaviors include flaccidity and a gape face (Als, 1986, 1996, 1997).

When the baby is organized and not stressed, the baby's **state and attention systems** are stable. The baby can move through clearly defined states of sleep, alertness, and crying. In the alert state, the baby can attend to and interact with the environment. When the baby is stressed, the sleep-wake cycles might be disturbed; crying and fussiness might be defined poorly; and inconsolability is common. The baby may use gaze aversion when stressed or make quick and unpredictable fluctuations between states instead of attending to and interacting with the environment (Als, 1986, 1996, 1997).

When the baby exhibits stress in any system, pay close attention to the signals, the behavioral language. The baby is communicating with you and asking you to modify what you are doing by changing your speed or direction of movement or choosing a novel toy. Sometimes you must stop what you are doing, comfort the baby, and help the baby recover a more organized, attentive state.

As already mentioned, the baby communicates through behavioral language and stress signals. When you learn to identify the baby's subtle language and stress signals and respond to them, you communicate back to the baby that you understand the message. If you miss the baby's subtle signals, they become more intense and sooner or later escalate to crying. In other words, crying often occurs because early signals of stress elude the caregiver. A baby who is crying is not in an optimal state to learn. The parents or caregivers of a crying baby also are stressed and not in an optimal state to learn. **Be intentional about learning babies' behavioral language so as to keep them from reaching the crying stage.**

Some babies will cry during therapy, but do not try to "push through" the baby's crying. Try to find the reason for the crying. Discuss the crying with the caregivers, and mutually decide on an approach to minimize it.

The baby communicates pleasure through smiles, eye contact, pleasant vocalizations, regulated breathing, stable color, and smooth participation with the activity. Be sure to acknowledge this communication and reciprocate with pleasant signals back to the baby.

Sensory Issues

We need sensory feedback in order to learn, regulate, and adapt our movements (Gordon, 1987; Cech & Martin, 1995). The visual, vestibular, and somatosensory systems are three primary systems through which we receive and channel sensory information. When sensory information coordinates with the motor system, we can make postural adjustments, perform movement, and learn and use motor skills.

Consequently, sensory input and feedback play a vital role in a baby's motor development. As the baby receives sensory information from the visual, vestibular, and somatosensory (tactile, proprioceptive, kinesthetic) systems, it is integrated with the motor system and enables the baby to adjust (right) the head, body, and limbs in space and in relation to each other and gravity (Shumway-Cook & Woollacott, 1995). The baby rights the head and trunk with extension in prone, flexes the head and trunk in supine, and laterally flexes the head and trunk in sidelying. In sitting and standing, the baby rights the head and trunk with extension when the center of mass shifts forward, with flexion when the center of mass shifts backward, and laterally when the center of mass shifts laterally.

Once the baby experiences and practices such movements and postural reactions, the baby learns to anticipate the need for the postural adjustments and subsequently makes the postural adjustments before the actual movement occurs. These adjustments—movements the baby makes in anticipation of the requirements and prior to sensory feedback—are called "feedforward" (Horak, 1991). In other words, we learn movements and postural adjustments through feedback and we then perform them with feedforward. We use feedforward in our habit patterns and "automatic" movements.

Because the baby learns movements and postural adjustments through sensory feedback, the baby must be able to receive, regulate, and adapt to this input to develop and perform optimally. The baby's reception of and adaptation to sensory feedback influences the movements the baby uses, the movements the baby practices, and the movements the baby learns and uses automatically with feedforward. A baby with sensory system impairments may learn, practice, and use compensatory or stereotyped movements habitually through feedforward. Small motor compensations early in development can lead to major motor-related problems in later life (Bly, 1983).

Some babies with motor problems have difficulty with reception, regulation, and/or adaptation to sensory stimuli. Some babies have "hyper" responses to sensory stimuli; others have "hypo" responses. Because the baby's early postural adjustments and movements are the foundation for future movements, early detection and treatment of sensory impairments are particularly important. Therefore, examination, evaluation, and treatment of the baby must include attention to the sensory systems.

You will enhance the baby's treatment when you determine if the baby's motor difficulties are the direct result of a motor impairment or an indirect result of a sensory impairment. For example, when a baby has poor head control, the baby's head is often in an abnormal position, i.e., the head lags when the baby is pulled to sit, or the head remains laterally tilted instead of adjusting to the vertical when the baby is sitting. Determining the source of the problem may be as simple as looking at the baby's facial expressions. If the baby does not seem to be stressed with the head in these positions, the baby may not be aware that the head is not in the optimal position. It is possible that the baby is not receiving or not processing the feedback that the head is not in an optimal position. In such occurrences, treatment must include techniques that enhance the sensory feedback in conjunction with the motor response.

On the other hand, if the baby's facial expression suggests that the baby is stressed and aware that the head is in an abnormal position, the baby's sensory feedback may be appropriate but the motor control may be ineffective in responding to the feedback. Treatment must include techniques that integrate the motor control with the sensory feedback.

In this text, sensory considerations accompany each illustrated facilitation technique. However, examination, evaluation, and treatment of serious sensory problems are beyond the scope and focus of this book. Further research on sensory topics is necessary (Blanche, Botticelli, & Hallway, 1995).

Kinesiological Issues

The baby's musculoskeletal system is incomplete in its development and is vulnerable to input and experiences. Consequently, the way the baby initially learns to move provides the kinesiological foundation for later movements.

Very young babies do not have full range of motion at all of their joints. Babies under 6 months of age often have limitations in spinal extension, hip extension, hip internal rotation, and shoulder flexion. (See Cusick, 1990, for more details on anatomical features of the lower extremities in infants.) Babies gradually increase the range of motion at each of their joints by practicing a variety of movements.

Babies typically activate and elongate their muscles by moving on all three planes of movement; sagittal, frontal, and transverse. They play with flexion and extension in supine; extension and flexion in prone; lateral weight shifts to each side in supine, prone, sitting, and standing; and rotation around the body axis in all positions. Flexion and extension occur on the sagittal plane; lateral movements, abduction, and adduction occur on the frontal plane; and rotation occurs on the transverse plane.

Babies with movement impairments do not practice movements on all three planes. They usually maintain a few positions and rarely alternate between positions. They often move primarily on the sagittal plane and subsequently develop stereotyped and compensatory movements. Because they do not use a variety of movement patterns, they have difficulty activating and elongating all of their muscles. Consequently, they may never develop full range of motion at all of their joints. If they do not develop full range of motion and do not elongate their muscles fully, they are vulnerable to musculoskeletal contractures and deformities.

The goals of the facilitation techniques in this book include **guiding** the baby through a variety of goal-directed movements to help the baby learn new movements. The facilitation techniques also help increase the baby's muscle extensibility and joint range of motion to prevent or minimize the development of musculoskeletal deformities. Try to select techniques that encourage the baby to alternate between positions, move on all three planes, and move through a variety of positions in each treatment session. The baby must be an active participant in the guided movements in order to take eventual control of the movements. You can help the baby to be an active participant by providing a motivating environment and helping the baby explore the environment.

Neutral alignment of body parts enables the muscles to work most efficiently. You can help the baby by providing neutral alignment of body parts when facilitating the baby through all of the different movements. When trying to align the baby's body parts, **never try to force** the baby into greater range of motion at any joint than is comfortable for the baby. If you are too aggressive, you can create a new skeletal impairment.

A common biomechanical problem recognized in older children with cerebral palsy is a kyphosis, flexion of the spine. The thoracic spine is especially vulnerable to this deformity. In order to prevent or minimize this problem, most of the facilitation techniques described in this book emphasize alignment and maintenance of alignment of the spine.

Another common biomechanical problem that occurs in older children with cerebral palsy is abnormal dissociation of the rib cage and pelvis: the rib cage moves over a stable pelvis, rather than the rib cage and pelvis moving synchronously. This often occurs because the thoracic spine has limited mobility in extension, lateral flexion, and rotation. Subsequently, the rib cage moves as unit, and hypermobility develops between the twelfth thoracic vertebra (T-12) and the first lumbar vertebra (L-1). In order to avoid this problem, the directions for the facilitation techniques always state to move the rib cage and pelvis sequentially, so that the pelvis moves over the femur at the hip joint. Do not rotate the rib cage over a stable pelvis.

Another progressive biomechanical problem frequently seen in older children with cerebral palsy is the "crouch-gait" posture, characterized by problems on all three planes. Foot pronation (dorsiflexion on the sagittal plane), eversion on the frontal plane, and abduction on the transverse plane can initiate this posture biomechanically. Excessive pronation can facilitate hip and knee flexion (a sagittal plane compensation), hip adduction (a frontal plane compensation), and hip internal rotation (a transverse plane compensation), which are the characteristics of the crouch gait.

The crouch-gait posture does not occur in the young baby because soft tissue tightness around the hip joints initially holds the hips in abduction, flexion, and external rotation. However, if therapy does not address the posture of the feet, the baby will develop these lower-extremity compensations over time. To prevent or minimize this problem when the baby bears weight on one or both feet, always transfer the weight to the lateral borders of the baby's feet. You can accomplish this by extending the baby's hip and knee and externally rotating the femur. If it is difficult to transfer the baby's weight to the lateral borders of the feet, the baby should wear orthotics.

Role of the Developmental Sequence

Historically, therapists used the developmental sequence as a model for therapeutic intervention, assuming that recovery after a neurological insult followed the same process as infant development (Gordon, 1987).

Designing or recommending treatment sequences that follow a developmental sequence is **not** the focus or intention of this book. I do not view the developmental sequence as a continuous process in which one milestone is the foundation for the next milestone. Instead, I view the milestones as age-appropriate behavioral characteristics (Bly, 1994).

However, in therapeutic work with babies, you should be intimately familiar with the developmental sequence, not to follow it but to establish age-appropriate goals for each baby. You need to know which motor skills the baby skipped or missed, which motor skills the baby should currently be engaged in, and which motor skills the baby should soon be engaged in.

Mary Quinton frequently stated that when treating a baby, one must work for the past, present, and future simultaneously (M. Quinton, personal lecture notes, 1976, 1978). A treatment session should include facilitation that addresses each condition, but not necessarily in a past-present-future order.

Ms. Quinton advised working "in the **past**" to fill up the gaps or holes in the baby's movement repertoire. When working "in the past," look for a common denominator that occurs in many of the problems, and continue to work on this until the baby uses it automatically.

Work "in the **present**" to enable the baby to participate in age-appropriate activities and to interact with self and caregivers. Remember, however, that the present quickly becomes the past when working with babies.

Work "in the **future**" to prepare the baby for age-appropriate activities of the future. It is important to work approximately 2 months ahead.

For example, a 7-month-old baby may have difficulty with weight shifts in sitting and therefore has difficulty moving into and out of sitting and difficulty with retrieving toys that are out of reach when sitting. Treatment of the **present** would include facilitated weight shifts through all planes of movement while sitting, facilitation of various transitions into and out of sitting, and use of toys that are motivating and easily controlled by the baby.

Further examination of the baby's skills may reveal that the baby also has difficulty with weight shifts in the prone position and a resultant inability to play with toys in prone. Most babies can shift weight in prone and play with toys with one hand by the age of 5 months. Therefore, treatment "of the **past**" for this 7-month-old baby could include facilitation of controlled weight shifts in prone and use of toys that are motivating and easily controlled by the baby. The therapist also could incorporate weight shifts in prone into transitions from prone to sitting.

To prepare this baby for the **future**, the therapist could facilitate the baby from sitting to standing and practice weight shifts in supported standing. Practicing weight shifts in standing helps prepare the baby for future walking.

In this example, the common denominator is the baby's poor ability to control lateral weight shifts. Therefore, the therapist would use facilitation techniques that include weight shifts throughout the treatment session. The order of the facilitation techniques can vary according to the baby's interests and desires. The session may begin in sitting and transition to the floor or to standing for a toy, then transition back to sitting. The session also may begin in prone or standing if preferred by the baby. Regardless of the order, the therapist can address the past, present, and future motor skills throughout the session.

Consider the past-present-future philosophy when planning and selecting facilitation techniques for the baby's treatment session.

Your Hands

Your hands **facilitate**, or assist, the baby through movements. Your hands guide the baby; they must never **push, pull, or force the baby.** Because of the size difference between you and the baby, it would be easy for you to overpower the baby's movements and take the baby through all of the facilitation techniques without the baby ever participating. That is never the goal of the facilitation.

Your hands align and maintain the alignment of the baby's body during the movement until the baby's own muscle control takes over. As the baby takes over the control for the alignment and the movement, you gradually reduce your control until you finally remove your hands. It is imperative that the baby take over the control. Therefore your hands must be sensitive to the baby's active participation.

When you are first learning the facilitation techniques, you probably will be more concerned with what you are doing than with what the baby is doing. The muscles in your hands (and probably your arms and body) will be working so hard that you will not be able to feel whether the baby's muscles are contracting. You are "fixing" or limiting your degrees of freedom. This is a normal process in motor learning. You must practice the facilitation techniques to reduce your fixing and become more sensitive to what the baby actually is doing. It is very helpful to practice with a rag doll. You **must** be sensitive to the baby's active control in order to modify your control and enable the baby to progress.

When you are facilitating, your *guiding hand* is the hand that controls the movement. Your *assisting hand* participates when the baby needs a little more help perform the movement smoothly and maintain proper alignment. Remember to wait for the baby to respond and participate. Your hands will feel this response after you become more comfortable with the techniques and you attend to the baby's responses.

Your hands communicate with the baby. They not only align the baby's body parts and tell the baby how to move; they also give the baby security and confidence. Your hands, along with your eyes, also detect how the baby is feeling. A baby who feels secure in your hands will let go of fixing patterns and participate in the movement. Your smiling face also is reassuring to the baby.

Play

Use of play is of vital importance when working with babies. Play is a functional activity in which all babies engage. It is their means to investigate and learn about the world. Their curiosity drives them to explore their world. This investigation introduces new motor challenges that necessitate problem solving and "research" into how to examine, manipulate, and use body parts, objects, other people, space, and sensory feedback effectively.

Play motivates the baby to move and learn new movement strategies; therefore, you will need to practice all of the facilitation techniques in the context of play. The movement itself and the sensory feedback from the movement may be exciting play to the baby. Play also may involve the use of toys.

When selecting toys for a baby, choose age-appropriate toys, even if the baby's motor skills are impaired. Babies often are disinterested or frustrated with toys that are below their age level. Select toys that will be interesting to the baby and enhance your treatment goals. Remember, it is important to permit the baby actually to play with the toy. Do not just use toys to distract the baby. Development of play skills is an important treatment goal.

Discovering and playing with body parts are important developmental steps for all babies. Babies explore their hands and feet with their eyes, hands, and mouths. Add these discoveries to your treatment sessions.

Music is motivating to many babies. You can use songs to engage a baby in specific movements. You don't even have to be able to carry a tune to engage the baby in the song. Music is also helpful in calming or alerting a baby.

It is important to find a play mode that will interest each baby. A baby who is not interested in play or does not know how to play often is not motivated to move. The baby's failing to participate actively in the movement will limit carryover and learning. It is critical that you find something that interests each baby because functional movement is goal-directed.

Equipment

You will perform the facilitation techniques on various pieces of equipment: your body, a ball, a bolster, or the floor. Try to use a variety of equipment, but when you select the equipment, consider whether you can manage both it and the baby simultaneously.

Use your body as equipment when the baby is small and fits easily on your lap or your legs. Your body can provide security to the baby because it is natural for babies to be held. Holding babies close to your body is especially important for babies who are insecure in open space.

Do not use your lap if the baby is too large. If the baby is too long for your lap and you try to flex the baby to work on the supine facilitation techniques, you will cause a thoracic kyphosis. This subsequently leads to neck hyperextension and all of the associated problems.

If you use your legs, your legs must be free to move up and down according to the baby's needs. When the baby is on your legs, your movements are very restricted. If you need to move or need to move the baby more freely, do not use your legs.

The bolster is the easiest piece of equipment to use because it moves on only one plane. Select a bolster that meets the baby's needs for height and width.

The ball is the most difficult piece of equipment to use because it is unpredictable and can roll anywhere. Larger balls are easier to manage than smaller balls because there is more surface area on which the baby can move. Use small balls if you want to transition the baby from the ball to the floor. Whichever ball you use, make sure that you are holding the baby securely so that if you lose control of the ball, you still have control of the baby.

The Family

The family members are obviously the most important people on the baby's team. Address the family's needs, support and encourage them, and educate and teach them about their baby's strengths as well as needs. Involve them immediately in planning the baby's treatment program, carrying over treatment activities, and setting goals for home. Feel free to give them as many treatment ideas as they can manage. The more involved the family becomes, the more consistent therapeutic management becomes for the baby. Treatment ideas that the family members can incorporate into the daily care of the baby will be easier to implement in the home setting.

Complex needs and stresses occur in families with a baby with special needs. Therapists, typically, have not been trained to deal with these issues. It is important for each of us to read and participate in workshops that teach us how to fit into the big picture so that we can be effective in helping support the baby and the family.

References

Als, H. (1986). A synactive model of neonatal behavioral organization: Framework for the assessment of neurobehavioral development in the premature infant and for support of infants and parents in the neonatal intensive care environment. In *The high-risk neonate: Developmental therapy perspectives.* In J. Sweeney (Ed.), *Physical and occupational therapy in pediatrics,* Vol. 6 (No. 3/4, pp. 3–53). Binghamton, NY: Halworth.

Als, H. (1996). Earliest intervention for preterm infants in the newborn intensive care unit. In M. J. Guralnick (Ed.), *The effectiveness of early intervention* (pp. 47–76). Baltimore: Paul H. Brookes.

Als, H. (1997). Neurobehavioral development of the preterm. In A. A. Fanaroff & R. J. Martin (Eds.), *Neonatal-perinatal medicine: Vol. 2.* (pp. 964–989). St. Louis, MO: C. V. Mosby.

Blanche, E., Botticelli, T., & Hallway, M. (1995). *Combining Neuro-Developmental Treatment and sensory integration principles.* San Antonio, TX: Therapy Skill Builders.

Bly, L. (1983). *The components of normal movement during the first year of life and abnormal motor development.* Monograph of the NDTA, 41–52.

Bly, L. (1994). *Motor skills acquisition in the first year: An illustrated guide to normal development.* San Antonio, TX: Therapy Skill Builders.

Bly, L., & Whiteside, A. (1997). *Facilitation techniques based on NDT principles.* San Antonio, TX: Therapy Skill Builders.

Cech, D., & Martin, S. (1995). *Functional movement development across the life span.* Philadelphia: W. B. Saunders.

Cusick, B. (1990). *Progressive casting and splinting for lower extremity deformities in children with neuromotor dysfunction.* San Antonio, TX: Therapy Skill Builders.

Gordon, J. (1987). Assumptions underlying physical therapy intervention: Theoretical and historical perspectives. In J. H. Carr, R. B. Shepherd, J. Gordon, A. M. Gentile, & J. M. Held (Eds.), *Movement science: Foundations for physical therapy in rehabilitation* (pp. 1–30). Rockville, MD: Aspen.

Horak, F. B. (1991). Assumptions underlying motor control for neurological rehabilitation. *Contemporary management of motor control problems: Proceedings of the II Step Conference,* American Physical Therapy Association, 11–27.

Shumway-Cook, A., & Woollacott, M. H. (1995). *Motor control.* Baltimore: Williams and Wilkins.

1. Supine

1.1 Visual Tracking

The goal of this facilitation is to check and facilitate the baby's visual tracking of a moving object. The baby should track the object horizontally and vertically. Facilitation of downward visual gaze is especially important because many babies with developmental delays have difficulty with symmetrical head flexion and subsequently have difficulty with visual convergence and downward movement of the eyes.

Additional goals include elongation of the spinal extensors, symmetrical activation of the neck and trunk flexors, activation of head movements in horizontal and vertical directions, and facilitation of active reaching.

Treatment of babies with severe visual problems is beyond the scope of this book.

Baby's Position The baby lies supine on the floor, an elevated mat, or your lap with the pelvis slightly elevated. **Do not overflex the baby's thoracic spine.**

Do not use your lap if you must overflex the baby's thoracic spine for the baby to fit on your lap. Use one of the other positions.

Therapist's Position
- Long-sit on the floor with the baby between your legs (figure 1.1.1). Capture the baby's visual gaze with an object. If it is difficult for the baby to maintain the head in the midline, abduct your hips and flex your knees so that your feet come together. Place a blanket or towel over your feet and rest the baby's head between your feet.
- Sit on the floor or a chair with the baby on your lap. Your hips must flex to at least 90° so that the baby's head and trunk are parallel with the floor and not tilting downward. Capture the baby's visual gaze with an object.
- If it is difficult to long-sit on the floor or to sit with the baby on your lap, place the baby on an elevated surface so you can stand during the technique. Capture the baby's visual gaze with an object.

Therapist's Hands and Movement Place both of your hands laterally on the baby's pelvis. Apply downward traction, lift the baby's pelvis slightly, and place it on your body. The traction elongates the baby's spinal extensors and the lifted pelvis maintains the elongation. **Do not flex the thoracic spine.**

Capture the baby's visual gaze with a high-contrast black and white toy (figure 1.1.1) or high-contrast primary color (red, blue, yellow) toy. Hold the object 10 to 12 inches from the baby's eyes.

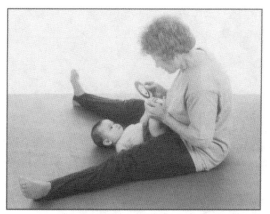

Figure 1.1.1. Visual tracking. The therapist long-sits on the floor with the baby lying supine between her legs, having lifted the baby's pelvis slightly to elongate the spinal extensors. The therapist uses a high-contrast object to attract the baby's gaze.

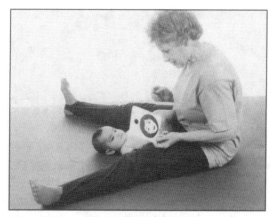

Figure 1.1.2. The therapist moves the object slowly from side to side.

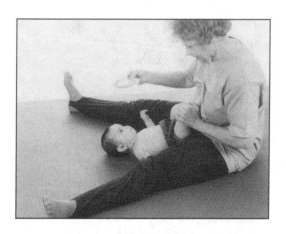

Figure 1.1.3. The therapist moves the object upward as far as the baby's vision follows in the baby's field of vision.

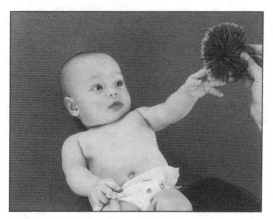

Figure 1.1.4. The therapist holds the toy to the side to encourage the baby to look to the side, locate the toy, and reach for it.

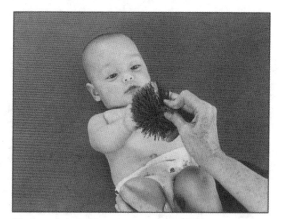

Figure 1.1.5. The therapist holds the toy in the midline and slightly down so as to encourage the baby to look down, locate the toy, and reach for it.

Once the baby looks at the object, move it slowly from side to side (figure 1.1.2), up (figure 1.1.3), and down (figure 1.1.1).

You also can hold the toy in one spot to encourage the baby to reach for the toy (figures 1.1.4, 1.1.5).

Precautions
- Do not flex the thoracic spine.
- Maintain the elevation of the pelvis.
- Move the toy slowly enough to maintain the baby's visual gaze.

Component Goals
- Activation of eye muscles
- Visual tracking
- Downward visual gaze
- Activation of head turning with rotation
- Activation of head, neck, and trunk flexors
- Activation of head extension and head flexion
- Elongation of spinal extensors, especially the cervical extensors
- Upper-extremity reaching

Functional Goals
- Moving of eyes for development of visual skills
- Activation of head movements for all movements
- Reaching in supine

1.2 Upper-Extremity Reaching for Self-Exploration With the Hands and Elongation of the Shoulder Girdle Muscles

The goal of these facilitation techniques is to elongate the scapulae and shoulder girdle muscles, enabling the baby to reach with each hand across the body to the opposite arm to explore the body. Additional goals include active elongation of the spinal extensors, symmetrical activation of the neck and trunk flexors, active shoulder flexion and elbow extension, tactile exploration with the hands, and hand shaping.

Baby's Position The baby lies supine on a mat, an elevated mat, or your lap with the pelvis slightly elevated. **Do not overflex the baby's thoracic spine.**

Do not use your lap if you must overflex the baby's thoracic spine for the baby to fit on your lap. Use one of the other positions.

Therapist's Position

- Long-sit on the floor with the baby between your legs (see figure 1.2.2). Capture the baby's visual gaze with your eyes.
- Sit on the floor or a chair with the baby on your lap. Your hips must flex to at least 90° so that the baby's head and trunk are parallel with the floor and not tilting downward. Capture the baby's visual gaze with your eyes.
- If it is difficult to long-sit on the floor or to sit with the baby on your lap, place the baby on an elevated surface so you can stand during the technique. Capture the baby's visual gaze with your eyes.

Therapist's Hands and Movement Place both of your hands laterally on the baby's trunk and pelvis (figure 1.2.1). Apply downward traction, lift the baby's pelvis slightly, and place it on or against your body. The traction elongates the baby's spinal extensors, and the lifted pelvis maintains the elongation. **Do not flex the thoracic spine.**

Note: The therapist in figure 1.2.1 is heel-sitting, but you can long-sit as you prepare the baby's posture.

Once you have elevated the baby's pelvis and elongated the spinal extensors, place both of your fingers firmly but gently on the baby's scapulae, with your thumbs lightly on the baby's humeri (figure 1.2.2).

While maintaining the gentle pressure, slowly abduct the baby's scapulae. As your hands get closer to the baby's humeri, use them to horizontally adduct the baby's arms as you maintain the pressure on the baby's scapulae (figure 1.2.2). You can put your face close to the baby's hands to encourage the baby to reach for your face. The baby's active reaching is very important and a goal of this facilitation technique.

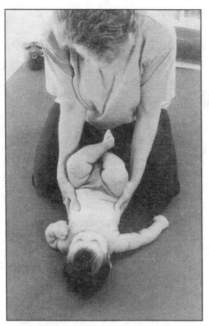

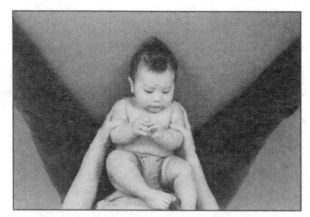

Figure 1.2.2. The therapist places the fingers of both hands on the baby's scapulae, thumbs lightly on the baby's humeri. Maintaining gentle pressure, the therapist slowly abducts the baby's scapulae and horizontally adducts the baby's arms.

Figure 1.2.1. Upper-extremity reaching. The therapist places both hands laterally on the baby's trunk and pelvis, then applies downward traction while lifting the baby's pelvis slightly to place it against the therapist's body.

Hands to Arms

Maintain the constant pressure and slowly slide your hands around the baby's shoulders and onto the baby's humeri. Use your hands to adduct one of the baby's arms gently onto the chest. Hold that arm on the baby's chest and continue to slide your hand along the baby's other arm with gentle traction until the baby's hand reaches the opposite arm (figure 1.2.3). Do not traction the baby's arm beyond the baby's comfort level. If the baby's hand comfortably reaches only to the chest, stop there.

Once the baby's hand reaches the opposite arm, move the reaching arm so that the baby's hand slides along the arm. The goal is to have the baby's hand open and gently grasp the arm. Continue to slide the open hand along the arm.

Maintain reassuring and smiling eye contact with the baby throughout the activity. Talk to the baby about the body as the baby touches specific body parts.

Repeat the facilitation with the opposite arm.

If the baby's shoulders elevate and the baby's neck hyperextends (the mouth also may open) during the facilitation (figure 1.2.4), use your index fingers to depress the shoulders gently (figure 1.2.5). This should elongate the neck extensors and enable the baby's head to flex (figure 1.2.5). Maintain the shoulder girdle depression as you adduct the baby's arm across the chest so that the baby's hand reaches the opposite arm (figure 1.2.6).

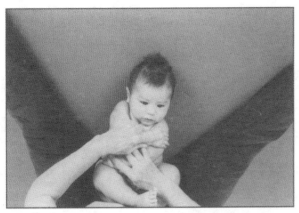

Figure 1.2.3. Hands to arms. Maintaining constant pressure, the therapist slides her hands around the baby's shoulders and onto the baby's humeri, gently adducting the baby's left arm onto the baby's chest. The therapist slides her left hand along the baby's right arm with gentle traction until the baby's right hand reaches the left arm.

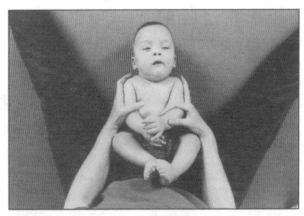

Figure 1.2.4. The baby's shoulders elevate, the neck hyperextends, and the mouth opens during the facilitation.

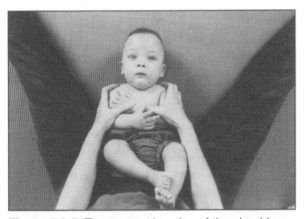

Figure 1.2.5. To counter elevation of the shoulders and hyperextension of the neck, the therapist uses index fingers to depress the baby's shoulders gently during the facilitation.

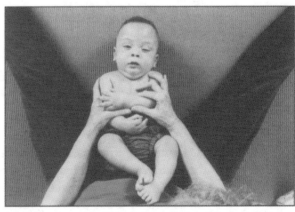

Figure 1.2.6. The therapist maintains the shoulder girdle depression while adducting the baby's arm across the chest so that the baby's hand reaches the opposite arm.

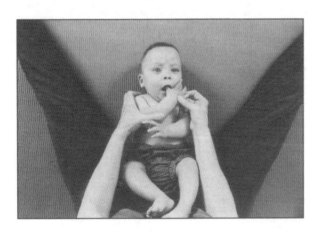

Figure 1.2.7. Hands to face and mouth. The therapist uses her fingers to maintain the baby's bilateral shoulder girdle depression and humeral adduction while using the thumb to guide the baby's elbow into flexion so that the baby's hand comes toward the face. Continuing to maintain the baby's opposite arm in adduction with the ulnar side of her other hand, the therapist uses her thumb and index finger to supinate the baby's forearm, open the baby's hand, and reach that hand to the opposite side of the baby's face. The baby's thumb ultimately goes in the baby's mouth.

Hands to Face and Mouth

Maintain the baby's bilateral shoulder girdle depression and humeral adduction with your fingers while you use your thumb to guide the baby's elbow into flexion so that the baby's hand comes toward the face (figure 1.2.7). While maintaining the baby's opposite arm in adduction with the ulnar side of your other hand, use your thumb and index finger to supinate the baby's forearm, open the baby's hand, and reach that hand to the opposite side of the face (figure 1.2.7). From this position, bring the baby's thumb to the mouth (figure 1.2.7). If the baby has teeth and/or a strong bite reflex, do not put the baby's thumb into the mouth. The baby's ability to bring the hand to the mouth will provide the baby with a means of self-comfort and self-consoling.

Repeat with the other hand.

Hand to Hand and Hands to Head

Continue to maintain the baby's humeri in adduction and slide your hands down to the baby's forearms (figure 1.2.8). Bring the baby's hands together and encourage the baby to look at the hands (figure 1.2.8). You can clap and/or rub the baby's hands together to get the baby's visual attention.

While holding the baby's forearms, gently flex the baby's shoulders so that the baby can reach the hands to the top of the head (figure 1.2.9). From this position of humeral flexion, carefully slide the baby's hands down across the face. You may do this unilaterally or bilaterally.

If the baby has hair and still has a grasp reflex, place your hand on the baby's head first, then place the baby's hand on your hand.

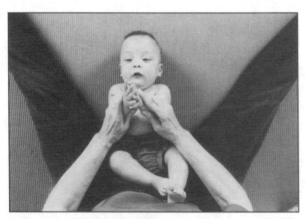

Figure 1.2.8. Hand to hand. The therapist continues to maintain the baby's humeri in adduction, sliding her hands down to the baby's forearms and bringing the baby's hands together while encouraging the baby to look at the hands.

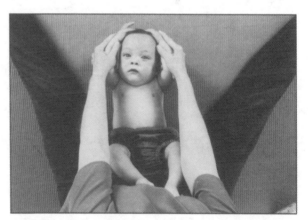

Figure 1.2.9. Hands to head. While holding the baby's forearms, the therapist gently flexes the baby's shoulders so the baby can reach the hands to the top of the head.

Precautions

- Do not flex the thoracic spine when elevating the baby's pelvis.
- Maintain the elevation of the pelvis.
- Abduct the baby's scapulae first.
- Do not pull the arms.
- If the baby resists the movement, reduce your pressure.
- Do not put the baby's hand in the mouth if the baby has a bite reflex.
- Place your hand over the baby's hair if the baby has a grasp reflex.

Component Goals

- Elongation of spinal extensors
- Activation of head, neck, and trunk flexors
- Elongation of scapulae adductors
- Elongation of scapulae elevators
- Elongation of humeral extensors
- Activation of humeral flexors and horizontal adductors
- Elongation of elbow flexors and forearm pronators
- Activation of elbow extensors and forearm supinators
- Hand-on-body play to decrease finger fisting and grasp reflex and increase active grasp with various shapes

Functional Goals

- Reaching of hands to various body parts for body awareness and body exploration
- Increased range of motion in shoulder girdles and upper extremities for all reaching patterns

1.3 Supine Flexion With Shoulder Girdle Depression

This technique works well in combination with the previous technique, or it may be used separately. You can use this facilitation with babies who maintain shoulder girdle elevation with strong contraction of the upper trapezius and levator scapulae muscles.

The goals of these facilitation techniques are for the baby to learn active symmetrical flexion in supine with depression of the shoulder girdles, elongation of neck and trunk extensors, and downward visual gaze.

Contraction of the upper trapezius and levator scapulae muscles facilitates scapular elevation and neck hyperextension and also may lead to an open mouth. In order for the baby to maintain the depression of the shoulder girdles, the baby must activate the abdominal and lower trapezius muscles.

Baby's Position The baby lies supine on the mat, or an elevated mat, with the pelvis slightly elevated. **Do not overflex the baby's thoracic spine.**

Therapist's Position

- Heel-sit on the floor so the baby's pelvis rests on your legs (see figure 1.3.3). You must be able to move with the baby. If you long-sit on the floor, you may not be able to shift your weight with the baby. Capture the baby's visual gaze with your eyes.
- If it is difficult to heel-sit on the floor, place the baby on an elevated mat so you can stand during the technique. Capture the baby's visual gaze with your eyes.

Suggestions for Infants Who Are Visually Impaired If the baby has a visual impairment, you will need to make adaptations to the visual component of the facilitation. For example, you may substitute auditory, tactile, vibratory, olfactory, or other stimuli for the visual stimuli. However, visual stimuli are the strongest and most age-appropriate stimuli.

Therapist's Hands and Movement Place your thumbs under the baby's knees and flex the baby's knees and hips. Then place the fingers of both of your hands laterally on the baby's trunk and pelvis (figure 1.3.1). Apply downward traction and lift the baby's pelvis slightly (figure 1.3.2) and place it on your body (figure 1.3.3). The traction elongates the baby's spinal extensors, and the lifted pelvis maintains the elongation. The elongation is most notable in the neck extensors as the baby's chin tucks. Do not flex the thoracic spine.

Note: Elongation of the baby's spinal extensors and lifting of the baby's pelvis can facilitate the baby to reach forward to the knees with the hands (figure 1.3.3).

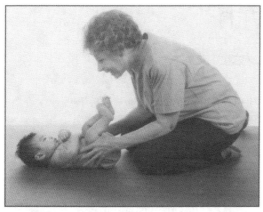

Figure 1.3.1. Supine flexion. The therapist places both thumbs under the baby's knees and flexes the baby's knees and hips, then places the fingers of both hands laterally on the baby's trunk and pelvis.

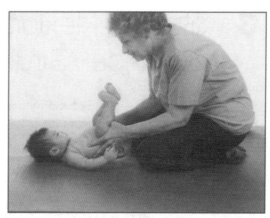

Figure 1.3.2. The therapist applies downward traction and lifts the baby's pelvis slightly.

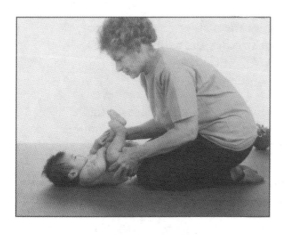

Figure 1.3.3. The therapist places the baby's pelvis on her knees. Elongation of the baby's spinal extensors and lifting of the baby's pelvis facilitates the baby to reach the hands forward to the knees.

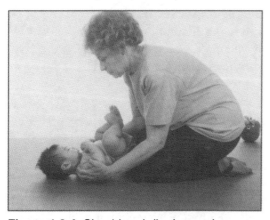

Figure 1.3.4. Shoulder girdle depression. Having placed her hands on the baby's scapulae, the therapist applies firm but gentle pressure with her hands and abducts the baby's scapulae. As the baby's scapulae abduct, the therapist slowly slides her hands around onto the baby's arms and brings them forward.

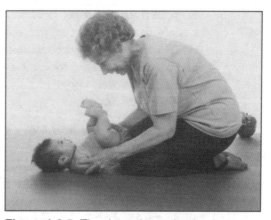

Figure 1.3.5. The therapist maintains her hands on the baby's arms, externally rotating them and applying slight downward traction to depress the baby's shoulders.

Shoulder Girdle Depression

Once you have elevated the baby's pelvis, carefully place your hands on the baby's scapulae. Apply firm but gentle pressure and abduct the baby's scapulae with your hands. As the baby's scapulae abduct, slowly slide your hands around onto the baby's arms and bring them forward (figure 1.3.4).

Maintain your hands on the baby's arms, externally rotate them, and apply slight downward traction to depress the baby's shoulders (figure 1.3.5). Maintain smiling eye contact with the baby. Your smiling face reassures the baby.

Hands to Hips

As the baby becomes comfortable with the shoulder depression (figure 1.3.5), maintain consistent contact with the baby's arms, applying slight traction while sliding your hands down the baby's arms (figure 1.3.6). Simultaneously press the baby's arms into the trunk. Continue to apply traction and slide your hands down the baby's arms until you can place the baby's hands on the hips (figure 1.3.6).

Once the baby's hands are on the hips, hold them there with your hands while you place your thumbs under the baby's thighs to maintain the hip flexion (figure 1.3.6). Remember to capture the baby's visual gaze with your smiling eyes and your face.

While stabilizing the baby in the flexed position (figure 1.3.6), roll the baby from side to side (figure 1.3.7). Remember to keep the baby's hips flexed, the pelvis elevated, and the arms adducted to the baby's sides.

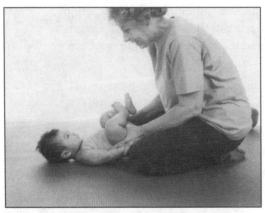

Figure 1.3.6. Hands to hips. Maintaining consistent contact with the baby's arms, the therapist applies slight traction and slides her hands down the baby's arms, simultaneously pressing the baby's arms into the trunk, until she can place the baby's hands on the hips. The therapist then holds the baby's hands on the hips with her hands while placing her thumbs under the baby's thighs to maintain the hip flexion.

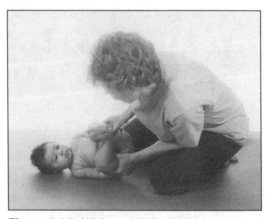

Figure 1.3.7. While stabilizing the baby in the flexed position, the therapist rolls the baby from side to side, shifting her weight and turning her head from side to side with the baby.

It is critical that you shift your weight and turn your head from side to side with the baby (figure 1.3.7). **You must maintain eye contact with the baby.** Frequently, it is the visual contact the baby has with you that facilitates the baby's head turning. When the baby rolls and turns the head actively with the body, the baby's abdominal muscles activate.

Option for Shoulder Girdle Depression

If the baby can accept and tolerate more specific elongation of the muscles that elevate the scapulae (levator scapulae and upper trapezius), place your hands directly on the baby's shoulders (figure 1.3.8).

Note: This initially may cause the baby to elevate the shoulders further. Maintain reassuring and smiling eye contact with the baby.

Align your index fingers with the baby's shoulders, and cup your hands around the baby's upper arms (figure 1.3.8). Carefully and slowly depress the baby's shoulders with your index fingers as you externally rotate and apply slight traction to the humeri with your hands (figure 1.3.9).

While maintaining the downward pressure with your index fingers and the traction with your hands, **gradually** increase the pressure to the shoulders while applying subtle vibrating movements to lower the shoulders further.

Shoulder depression should result in elongation of the baby's neck and subtle head and neck flexion (figure 1.3.9). As you depress the baby's shoulders, use your ulnar-side fingers to assist the baby to bring the arms forward.

The baby's pelvis must remain elevated to elongate the head and neck extensors.

Once you have depressed the baby's shoulders, maintain the depression and slide your hands down the baby's arms until the baby's hands rest on the baby's hips. Roll the baby from side to side to activate the baby's flexor muscles.

Note: Many babies will not accept this method of elongating the muscles that elevate the scapulae. Do not use this technique with these babies.

Precautions

- Do not flex the thoracic spine when elevating the baby's pelvis.
- Maintain the elevation of the pelvis.
- Maintain reassuring and smiling eye contact with the baby through the entire facilitation.
- Never cause pain to the baby. If the baby resists the movement, reduce your pressure.
- Carefully depress the baby's shoulders. Do not force the movement.
- Gradually increase your pressure and traction to the baby's arms.
- Maintain the baby's hips in flexion and keep the pelvis elevated while rolling the baby from side to side.
- You must shift your weight and turn your head from side to side with the baby.

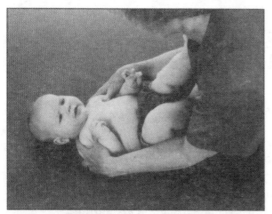

Figure 1.3.8. Option for shoulder girdle depression. The therapist places her hands directly on the baby's shoulders, aligning her index fingers with the baby's shoulders and cupping her hands around the baby's upper arms.

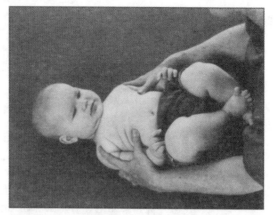

Figure 1.3.9. The therapist carefully and slowly depresses the baby's shoulders with her index fingers as she externally rotates and applies slight traction to the humeri with her hands.

Component Goals

- Elongation of spinal extensors
- Elongation of hip extensors
- Activation of head, neck, trunk, hip, and knee flexors
- Symmetrical flexion of head, neck, and trunk
- Elongation of scapulae elevators
- Active head turning
- Visual tracking
- Self-exploration
- Hands shaping to body parts

Functional Goals

- Increased range of motion in head-neck-shoulder girdle muscles for development of head control
- Increased range of motion in shoulder girdles and upper extremities for all reaching patterns
- Activation of abdominal muscles to stabilize the thorax for head and upper-extremity movements
- Visual tracking for eye muscle development

1.4 Tactile and Visual Body Exploration With Hands and Eyes

The goal of this facilitation technique is to enable the baby to use tactile and visual feedback, exploring body parts to increase body awareness. Additional goals include elongation of the spinal extensors, symmetrical activation of the neck and trunk flexors, facilitation of active reaching and grasping, and activation of downward visual gaze and gaze shifting.

Baby's Position The baby lies supine on the mat, an elevated mat, or your lap with the pelvis slightly elevated. **Do not overflex the baby's thoracic spine.**

Do not use your lap if you must overflex the baby's thoracic spine for the baby to fit on your lap. Use one of the other positions.

Therapist's Position

- Heel-sit on the floor in front of the baby. Capture the baby's visual gaze with your eyes.
- Sit on the floor or a chair with the baby on your lap. Your hips must flex to at least 90° so that the baby's head and trunk are parallel with the floor and not tilting downward. Lap-sitting is especially nice but works only with very small babies. Capture the baby's visual gaze with your eyes.
- If it is difficult to long-sit on the floor or to sit with the baby on your lap, place the baby on an elevated surface so you can stand during the technique. Capture the baby's visual gaze with your eyes.

Therapist's Hands and Movement Place both of your hands laterally on the baby's trunk and pelvis (see figure 1.2.1). Apply downward traction, lift the baby's pelvis slightly, and place it on your body. The traction elongates the baby's spinal extensors, and the lifted pelvis maintains the elongation. **Do not flex the thoracic spine.**

You may use this initial movement for each of the following techniques, or you may choose the optional initial movements.

Hand to Hand

Once you have elevated the baby's pelvis and elongated the spinal extensors, cup your hands around the baby's arms and bring them forward so that the baby's hands come together (see figure 1.2.8 on page 17). Encourage the baby to look at the hands. You can clap and/or rub the baby's hands together to get the baby's visual attention. If the baby accomplishes this goal, stay in this position, play with the baby's hands, and encourage the baby to look down to the hands.

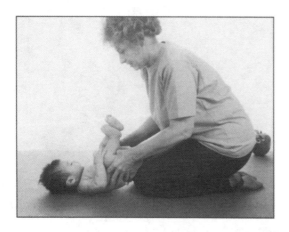

Figure 1.4.1. Tactile and visual body exploration with hands and eyes: Hands to knees. The therapist places both hands laterally on the baby's trunk and pelvis, with thumbs under the baby's thighs. The therapist flexes the baby's hips with her thumbs as she applies downward traction with her hands, lifts the baby's pelvis slightly, and places it on her body. The therapist encourages the baby to play with the hands on the knees, incorporating the baby's vision with the activity.

From this position, you can rub the baby's hand along the baby's arm and encourage visual following of the hand.

Maintain reassuring and smiling eye contact with the baby throughout the activity.

Suggestion Keep the baby in this position while you apply cream to the baby's body. This will provide additional tactile stimuli.

Hands to Knees

Place both of your hands laterally on the baby's trunk and pelvis with your thumbs under the baby's thighs (figure 1.4.1). Flex the baby's hips with your thumbs as you apply downward traction with your hands, then lift the baby's pelvis slightly and place it on your body. The traction elongates the baby's spinal extensors, and the lifted pelvis maintains the elongation. **Do not flex the thoracic spine.**

Once you have elevated the baby's pelvis, maintain the traction on the trunk and keep the baby's hips flexed. Stay in this position and encourage the baby to play with the hands on the knees. Incorporate the baby's vision with the activity. This is an especially good position for activating the baby's downward vision as the baby looks at the hands and the knees (figure 1.4.1).

You may shift the baby's weight slowly from side to side. The weight shifts should be subtle and should not disturb the baby's play.

Maintain reassuring and smiling eye contact with the baby throughout the activity.

Hands to Legs

Optional Initial Movement Place one hand posteriorly on the baby's pelvis and apply downward traction while lifting the pelvis slightly from the floor (figure 1.4.2). **Do not flex the thoracic spine.**

Once you have applied traction and elevated the baby's pelvis, maintain the traction on the trunk with one hand and place your other hand on the baby's legs to guide them into flexion. Flex the baby's legs until they

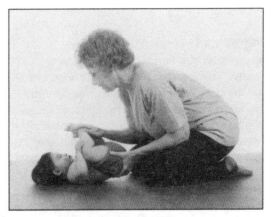

Figure 1.4.2. Hands to legs. The therapist applies downward traction to elevate the baby's pelvis, then maintains the traction on the trunk with one hand and places her other hand on the baby's legs, guiding them into flexion until they come into the baby's visual field.

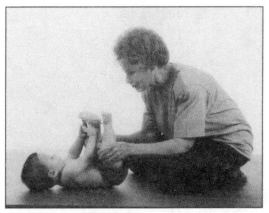

Figure 1.4.3. Hands to feet. The therapist places both of her hands on the baby's legs near the knees, with thumbs under the knees. The therapist flexes the baby's hips and lifts the pelvis slightly from the floor, then plays with the baby's hands on the legs and feet, activating the baby's visual gaze shifting as the baby looks from one foot to the other.

come into the baby's visual field. Do not force the baby's legs into flexion. If the baby resists, reduce your pressure.

Stay in this position and encourage the baby to play with the hands on the legs. Wait for the baby to look at the hands and the legs; this incorporates the baby's vision into the activity. This is an especially good position to activate the baby's downward vision as the baby looks at the hands and the legs (figure 1.4.2).

You may shift the baby's weight slowly from side to side. The weight shifts should be subtle and should not disturb the baby's play.

Maintain reassuring and smiling eye contact with the baby throughout the activity.

Hands to Feet

Optional Initial Movement Place both of your hands on the baby's legs near the knees. Place your thumbs under the knees (figure 1.4.3).

Flex the baby's hips and lift the pelvis slightly from the floor (figure 1.4.3). While keeping the baby's hips flexed, you may apply slight downward traction to the baby's trunk to elongate the spinal extensors. **Do not flex the thoracic spine.**

Stay in this position and play with the baby's hands on the legs and feet. Make sure that the baby looks at the hands and the feet; this incorporates vision into the activity. This is an especially good position for activating the baby's visual gaze shifting as the baby looks from one foot to the other (figure 1.4.3).

Maintain reassuring and smiling eye contact with the baby throughout the activity.

Precautions

- Do not flex the thoracic spine.
- Maintain the elevation of the pelvis.
- Do not force any movement. If the baby resists the movement, reduce your pressure.

Component Goals

- Elongation of spinal extensors
- Activation of head, neck, and trunk flexors
- Shoulder flexion with elbow extension
- Hip flexion with knee flexion
- Hip flexion with knee extension
- Hand-on-body play to decrease grasp reflex and increase active grasp with various shapes
- Downward visual gaze
- Purposeful shifting of visual gaze

Functional Goals

- Reaching of hands and vision to various body parts for body awareness and body exploration
- Reaching in supine
- Eye movement for development of visual skills

1.5 Supine to Sit

The goal of this facilitation is to bring the baby to sitting so the baby can learn to go to sitting independently.

Baby's Position The baby lies supine on the mat or an elevated mat (figure 1.5.1).

Therapist's Position

- Heel-sit on the floor in front of the baby and engage the baby visually (figure 1.5.1).
- Stand in front of the baby if the baby is on an elevated mat.

Therapist's Hands and Movement Place both of your hands on the baby's trunk. Slowly rotate the baby's rib cage and pelvis to one side so that the baby can push up on one hand (figure 1.5.2). Stay in this

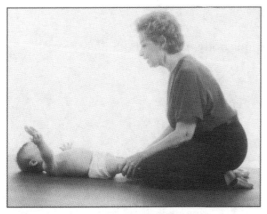

Figure 1.5.1. Supine to sit. With the baby lying supine on the mat, the therapist heel-sits in front of the baby and engages the baby visually.

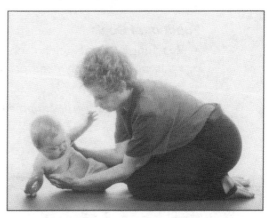

Figure 1.5.2. The therapist places both hands on the baby's trunk, then slowly rotates the baby's rib cage and pelvis to one side so that the baby can push up on one hand.

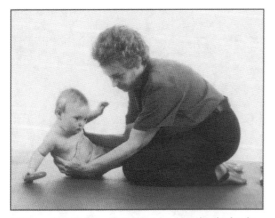

Figure 1.5.3. The therapist keeps the baby in the rotated position until the baby's head moves into a position of lateral righting.

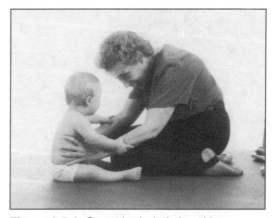

Figure 1.5.4. Once the baby's head has righted, the therapist continues the transition up to sitting, using both hands to stabilize the baby's trunk once the baby is in the sitting position.

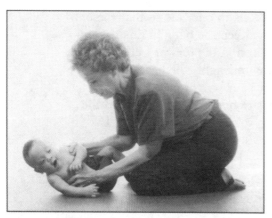

Figure 1.5.5. Option if the baby uses strong scapular adduction and humeral extension on the unweighted side. The therapist places her hand on the baby's scapula and arm, brings the baby's arm forward onto the baby's chest, and holds it there, placing her other hand on the baby's trunk to control the rib cage. The therapist then slowly rotates the baby's rib cage and pelvis to one side so that the baby can push up on one hand.

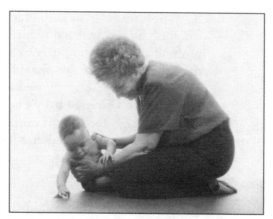

Figure 1.5.6. The therapist maintains the baby in this rotated position with the baby's back arm in the forward position until the baby bears weight on the other arm and rights the head.

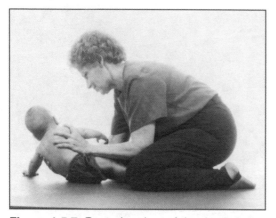

Figure 1.5.7. Posterior view of the therapist's hands stabilizing the baby's trunk and the back arm in a forward position as the therapist rotates the baby's trunk.

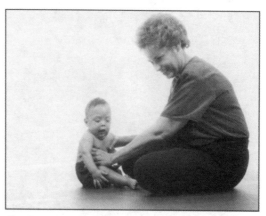

Figure 1.5.8. Once the baby's head has righted, the therapist continues to hold the arm forward as the baby transitions up to sitting.

rotated position until the baby's head moves into a position of lateral righting (figure 1.5.3). This will indicate that the baby is participating actively in the transition. Once the baby's head has righted, continue the transition up to sitting (figure 1.5.4). Use both of your hands to stabilize the baby's trunk once the baby is in the sitting position.

Option If the baby uses strong scapular adduction and humeral extension on the unweighted side, place your hand on the baby's scapula and arm and bring the baby's arm forward onto the baby's chest and hold it there (figure 1.5.5). Place your other hand on the baby's trunk to control the rib cage.

Slowly rotate the baby's rib cage and pelvis to one side so that the baby can push up on one hand (figure 1.5.5). Keep the baby in this rotated position and maintain the baby's back arm in the forward position until the baby bears weight on the other arm and rights the head (figures 1.5.6 and 1.5.7). You will need to shift your weight as the baby's weight shifts. Once the baby's head has righted, continue to hold the arm forward as the baby transitions up to sitting (figure 1.5.8). Use both of your hands to stabilize the baby's trunk once the baby is in the sitting position.

Component Goals

- Rotation of the trunk and pelvis over the hip
- Upper-extremity weight bearing
- Lateral righting of the head
- Oblique abdominal activation

Functional Goals

- Independent transition from supine to sitting
- Upper-extremity propping to prevent a fall from the sitting position

2. Supine Rolling

The goals of these techniques are to help the baby learn to play in flexion when in supine and to roll from supine to sidelying and to prone.

Babies who are developing typically usually do not like supine after the sixth or seventh month of life. They prefer to roll to prone and play. In the supine position, babies are very limited in what they can do. They can reach out to dangling toys and hold and finger very light toys. They cannot explore the world from the supine position. Therefore, you should use the supine facilitation techniques described in this book primarily for babies who are 7 months or younger. Of course, there are always exceptions to this suggestion.

2.1 Hands to Feet: Symmetrical Rolling

The goals of this facilitation are for the baby to learn to reach the hands to the feet, symmetrical trunk flexion, and symmetrical rolling in supine. Additional goals include elongation of the spinal extensors, hip extensors, and knee flexors; activation of the neck, trunk, and shoulder flexors; and activation of visual gaze to the feet and hands.

Baby's Position The baby lies supine on the mat, with the hips and knees flexed. If the baby's legs are extended on the mat, choose one of the following options.

- Elevate the baby's pelvis and place it on your body. This should facilitate the baby's hip and knee flexion.
- Begin the technique by placing your thumbs under the baby's ankles. Flex the baby's hips, and bring the baby's legs to the baby's hands.

Therapist's Position Heel-sit in front of the baby in a position to move with the baby. It is important that you capture the baby's visual gaze with your eyes.

If it is difficult to heel-sit, place the baby on an elevated mat so you can stand during the technique.

Therapist's Hands and Movement Once you have lifted the baby's pelvis, place your hands on the baby's legs near the ankles. Move the baby's legs toward the baby's hands. While holding the baby's legs, place your index fingers in the palms of the baby's hands (figure 2.1.1). Wrap your other fingers around the baby's hands and hold them and the baby's legs securely. You may have to reach for one hand at a time.

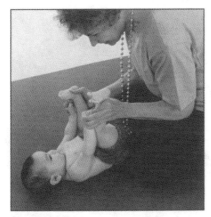

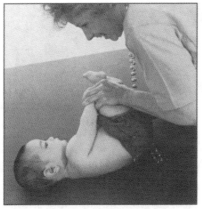

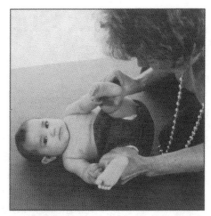

Figure 2.1.1. Hands to feet: Symmetrical rolling. The therapist lifts the baby's pelvis, places her hands on the baby's legs near the ankles, then moves the baby's legs toward the baby's hands. While holding the baby's legs, the therapist places her index fingers in the palms of the baby's hands and wraps her other fingers around the baby's hands, holding them and the baby's legs securely.

Figure 2.1.2. Holding the baby's visual gaze with her eyes and the baby's hands and legs **with the pelvis elevated,** the therapist moves her head to the side while simultaneously applying traction to the arm and leg on the baby's soon-to-be unweighted side so the arm and leg reach across the baby's body. The therapist continues the traction and head movement until the baby rolls symmetrically to the side.

Figure 2.1.3. The therapist repeats the movement to the other side.

While holding the baby's hands and legs, return the baby to the midline and lift the baby's pelvis sufficiently to elongate the neck and trunk extensors, but do not flex the baby's thoracic spine (figure 2.1.1). Capture the baby's visual gaze with your eyes.

While holding the baby's visual gaze with your eyes and the baby's hands and legs **with the pelvis elevated,** move your head to the side while simultaneously applying traction to the arm and leg on the baby's soon-to-be unweighted side so that the arm and leg reach across the baby's body (figure 2.1.2). Continue the traction and your head movement until the baby rolls symmetrically to the side. The baby's head must turn symmetrically with the body. Repeat the movement to the other side (figure 2.1.3). Shift the baby's weight from side to side several times.

Suggestion Wear a bright necklace around your neck to capture the baby's visual attention.

Option If the baby can reach actively for the feet, use your hands to apply downward traction to the pelvis and trunk while you slightly lift the pelvis (figure 2.1.4). Place the baby's feet into the baby's visual field. Wait for the baby to reach the hands to the feet (figure 2.1.4).

Once the baby reaches for the feet, slide your hands up on the baby's legs so that you can reach your index fingers to the baby's arms to stabilize them as you assist the baby to roll to the side (figure 2.1.5).

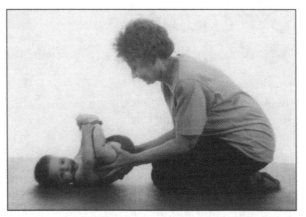

Figure 2.1.4. Option for a baby who can reach actively for the feet. The therapist uses her hands to apply downward traction to the pelvis and trunk while slightly lifting the pelvis. The therapist then places the baby's feet into the baby's visual field and waits for the baby to reach the hands to the feet.

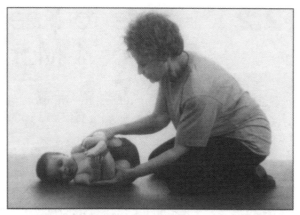

Figure 2.1.5. Once the baby reaches for the feet, the therapist slides her hands up on the baby's legs, reaching index fingers to the baby's arms to stabilize them while assisting the baby to roll to the side.

Precautions

- Do not flex the baby's thoracic spine. Keep the baby's trunk straight as you lift the baby's pelvis.
- Maintain the elevation of the pelvis. If you lower the pelvis, the baby's neck will hyperextend, followed by trunk hyperextension.
- Maintain the baby's visual gaze with your visual gaze to facilitate downward vision and head turning with the trunk. Encourage the baby's interests in the feet to maintain the downward visual gaze.

Component Goals

- Elongation of the spinal extensors
- Activation of the neck and trunk flexors (abdominals)
- Hip flexion with knee extension
- Shoulder flexion with active reaching
- Activation of downward visual gaze
- Sensory feedback (tactile, vestibular, proprioceptive, and visual) of sidelying to facilitate lateral righting reactions

Functional Goals

- Reaching with the hands and vision to the feet for body exploration
- Downward visual gaze for body exploration
- Independent rolling from supine to sidelying

2.2 Hands-to-Knees Symmetrical Rolling: 4-Month Roll

This technique is an imitation of how the 4-month-old baby typically reaches hands to knees and rolls from supine to sidelying and back again.

The goals of this facilitation are for the baby to learn symmetrical flexion in supine by reaching the hands to the knees and to learn to roll from side to side in this position. Additional goals include elongation of the spinal extensors; activation of the neck, trunk, and shoulder flexors; and activation of downward visual gaze.

Baby's Position The baby lies supine on the mat, with the hips and knees flexed (figure 2.2.1).

If the baby's legs are extended on the mat, choose one of the following options.

- Elevate the baby's pelvis and place it on your body. This should facilitate the baby's hip and knee flexion.
- Begin the technique by placing your thumbs under the baby's knees. Flex the baby's knees and bring them to the baby's hands.

Therapist's Position Heel-sit in front of the baby in a position to move with the baby (figure 2.2.1). It is important that you capture the baby's visual gaze with your eyes.

If it is difficult to heel-sit, place the baby on an elevated mat so you can stand during the technique.

Therapist's Hands and Movement Extend your index fingers into the baby's visual field so that the baby sees your fingers and reaches for them (see figure 2.3.1). If the baby does not reach for your fingers, provide tactile stimulation to facilitate the reach by sliding your index fingers gently on the baby's arms (figure 2.2.1). Move your fingers from proximal to distal, bringing your fingers into the palms of the baby's hands (figure 2.2.2). As the baby clasps your fingers, wrap your other fingers around the baby's wrists, hold them securely, and bring the baby's hands to the baby's knees (figure 2.2.3).

Place your thumbs under the baby's knees to hold the knees and hips in flexion (figure 2.2.3).

From this flexed position, roll the baby symmetrically to the side (figure 2.2.4). The baby's head must turn actively and follow the body; therefore, you must keep the baby's visual attention and turn your head with the baby's weight shift.

Remember to keep the baby's pelvis elevated. If the baby tries to extend the neck, elevate the pelvis a little higher but do not flex the thoracic spine.

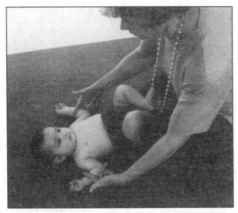

Figure 2.2.1. Hands-to-knees symmetrical rolling: 4-month roll. With the baby in supine on the mat with the hips and knees flexed, the therapist slides her index fingers gently on the baby's arms to provide tactile stimulation to facilitate the reach.

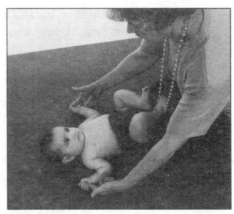

Figure 2.2.2. The therapist moves her index fingers along the baby's arms from proximal to distal, ending in the palms of the baby's hands.

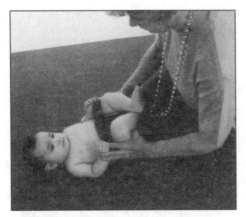

Figure 2.2.3. As the baby clasps the therapist's fingers, the therapist wraps her other fingers around the baby's wrists, holds them securely, and brings the baby's hands to the baby's knees. The therapist then places her thumbs under the baby's knees to hold the knees and hips in flexion.

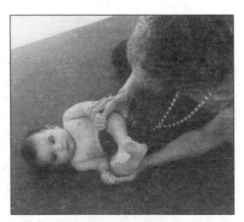

Figure 2.2.4. The therapist rolls the baby symmetrically to the side. The baby's head must turn actively and follow the body.

Remain in the Sidelying Position

Once the baby has rolled to the side, stay in the sidelying position for a few seconds so that the baby accommodates to the sensory stimuli of this position. If the baby is uncomfortable in the sidelying position, remain in that position only briefly but continue to come back to the position in order for the baby to adapt to the position and the sensory stimuli.

When rolling from supine to sidelying, there is a change in the stimuli to the visual, vestibular, tactile, proprioceptive, and auditory systems.

The baby must learn to adjust and accommodate to the changing feedback from each of these systems.

Return to Midline
Return the baby to midline from the sidelying position and remain there for a few seconds. Try to capture the baby's visual attention and position your face so that the baby's eyes gaze downward.

Roll to the Other Side
Roll the baby symmetrically to the other side and stay there for a few seconds. Roll the baby slowly and deliberately from side to side several times.

Do not roll the baby quickly. Allow the baby time to adjust to the movement and the different positions.

Precautions
- Do not flex the baby's thoracic spine. Keep the baby's trunk straight as you lift the baby's pelvis.
- Maintain the elevation of the pelvis. If you lower the baby's pelvis, the baby's neck will hyperextend, followed by trunk hyperextension.
- Do not move quickly.
- Allow the baby time to adjust to the sidelying positions.
- Do not force the baby to remain in sidelying for a long time if the baby appears to be uncomfortable in that position.
- Maintain the baby's visual gaze with your visual gaze to facilitate downward vision and head turning with the trunk.

Component Goals
- Elongation of the spinal extensors
- Activation of the neck and trunk flexors (abdominals)
- Hip and knee flexion
- Shoulder flexion with active reaching
- Activation of downward visual gaze
- Sensory feedback of sidelying to facilitate lateral righting reactions

Functional Goals
- Reaching hands to knees for body exploration
- Downward visual gaze for body exploration
- Independent rolling from supine to sidelying
- Adjustment and adaptation of the sensory systems (visual, vestibular, tactile, proprioceptive, kinesthetic, and auditory) to the changing feedback

2.3 Hands-to-Knees Roll to Asymmetrical Sidelying: 5-Month Roll

This technique is a modification of how the 5-month-old baby typically rolls from supine to sidelying and back again. You can use this technique as a continuation of the previous technique, 4-Month Roll.

The goal of this facilitation is for the baby to learn to roll from symmetrical flexion in supine to sidelying with lateral flexion and lower-extremity dissociation. Additional goals include elongation of the weight-bearing side, lateral righting of the unweighted side, and upper-extremity dissociation.

Baby's Position The baby lies supine on the mat.

Therapist's Position Heel-sit in front of the baby in a position to move with the baby (figure 2.3.1). It is important that you capture the baby's visual gaze with your eyes.

If it is difficult to heel-sit, place the baby on an elevated mat so that you can stand during the technique.

Therapist's Hands and Movement Extend your index fingers into the baby's visual field so that the baby becomes interested in them and reaches for them (figure 2.3.1). (You can stay in this position, play with the baby's hands, and encourage the baby to look down to the hands.)

As the baby reaches for your hands, place your index fingers in the baby's palms. Wrap your other fingers around the baby's hands or

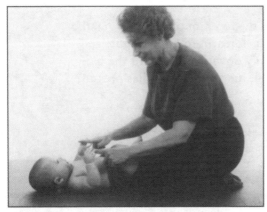

Figure 2.3.1. Hands-to-knees roll to asymmetrical sidelying: 5-month roll. The therapist heel-sits in front of the baby in a position to move with the baby and extends her index fingers into the baby's visual field so that the baby becomes interested in them and reaches for them.

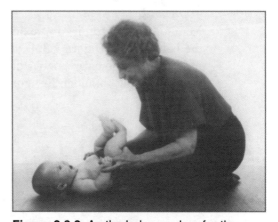

Figure 2.3.2. As the baby reaches for the therapist's hands, the therapist places her index fingers in the baby's palms, wraps her other fingers around the baby's wrists, and holds them securely. The therapist brings the baby's hands toward the baby's knees, places her thumbs under the baby's knees, and flexes the baby's knees and hips.

wrists and hold them securely (figure 2.3.2). Bring the baby's hands toward the baby's knees, place your thumbs under the baby's knees, and flex the baby's knees and hips (figure 2.3.2).

This position is similar to the typical 4-month position of hands to knees. From this flexed position, the baby learns to roll to the side and eventually learns to roll to prone.

Options

If the baby's legs are extended when you initiate this technique, choose one of the following options to flex the baby's legs.

- Elevate the baby's pelvis and place it on your body. This should facilitate the baby's hip and knee flexion. With the baby's pelvis resting on your body, place your index fingers into the baby's palms. Wrap your other fingers around the baby's hands or wrists and hold them securely (figure 2.3.2). Bring the baby's hands toward the baby's knees, place your thumbs under the baby's knees, and flex the baby's knees and hips (figure 2.3.2).

- Begin the technique by placing your thumbs under the baby's knees. Flex the baby's knees and hips. Continue to flex the baby's hips until you can place your index fingers into the baby's palms (figure 2.3.2).

Symmetrical Roll to the Side

Once you have elevated the baby's pelvis and elongated the spinal extensors, maintain your hand position and roll the baby symmetrically to one side (figure 2.3.3).

Make sure that you shift your weight with the baby (figure 2.3.3).

5-Month Position

Once the baby has rolled to the side, continue to maintain the baby's pelvis in the elevated position with both of your hands. Place the forearm of your top hand on the baby's pelvis (figure 2.3.4).

Top Hand

Maintaining the top leg in flexion and the forearm of your top hand on the baby's pelvis (figure 2.3.4), use your forearm to apply **slight** pressure into the baby's pelvis diagonally downward toward the baby's weight-bearing shoulder. In figure 2.3.4, the therapist applies pressure

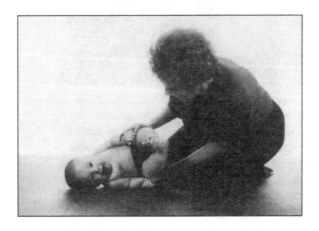

Figure 2.3.3. Symmetrical roll to the side. The therapist maintains her hand position and rolls the baby symmetrically to one side, shifting her weight with the baby.

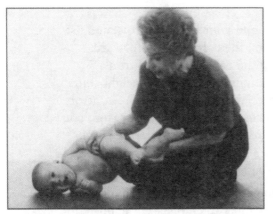

Figure 2.3.4. 5-month position. The therapist maintains the top leg in flexion and places the forearm of her top hand on the baby's pelvis, using her forearm to apply slight pressure into the baby's pelvis, diagonally downward toward the baby's weight-bearing shoulder. The therapist has released the baby's bottom hand but continues to hold the baby's bottom leg, using her bottom hand to apply traction simultaneously to the baby's lower leg to extend the lower hip and knee and lift the pelvis.

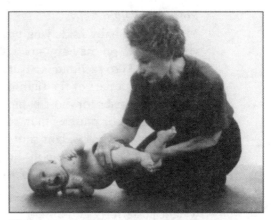

Figure 2.3.5. The therapist maintains the baby's sidelying position and hand controls, using her forearm on the baby's pelvis to roll the baby slightly forward to facilitate activation of the baby's neck and trunk extensors.

from the left side of the baby's pelvis diagonally down to the baby's right shoulder.

If the baby does not try to retract the top arm, you can let go of the baby's top hand (figure 2.3.5).

Bottom Hand
Once the baby is in sidelying, release the baby's bottom hand but continue to hold the baby's bottom leg (figure 2.3.4).

Both Hands
While stabilizing the baby's pelvis with your top arm, use your bottom hand to apply traction simultaneously to the baby's lower leg to extend the lower hip and knee and lift the pelvis (figure 2.3.4). Do not force the extension. If the baby resists lower-extremity extension, reduce your pressure but do not let go entirely.

The traction and lifting of the baby's bottom leg and the slight diagonally downward pressure through the baby's pelvis facilitate lateral flexion of the baby's neck and trunk.

Backward Weight Shifts
Maintain the baby's sidelying position and your hand controls, and use your forearm on the baby's pelvis to roll the baby slightly backward to facilitate activation of the baby's neck and trunk flexors as a part of the righting reactions. Most babies need to experience the backward weight shifts frequently to activate their abdominal muscles. (Note the difference in the baby's face, eyes, and mouth in figures 2.4.3, 2.4.4, and 2.4.5. In figure 2.4.4, the baby's weight has shifted posteriorly.)

Forward Weight Shifts

Maintain the baby's sidelying position and your hand controls, and use your forearm on the baby's pelvis to roll the baby slightly forward (figure 2.3.5) to facilitate activation of the baby's neck and trunk extensors as a part of the righting reactions. The forward weight shifts usually are easier for most babies, especially if they have more control of their extensor muscles than their flexor muscles. For this reason, you should use forward weight shifts less frequently than posterior weight shifts. (Note the extension in the baby's head and trunk in figure 2.4.5 when the therapist shifts the baby's weight forward.)

Stay in the elongated sidelying position and alternately shift the baby's weight posteriorly and anteriorly. Remember to emphasize the posterior weight shifts more than the anterior weight shifts for most babies.

Symmetry

Use both of your hands to maintain the elevated position of the baby's pelvis and return the baby to symmetrical supine. You do not have to hold the baby's hands after the initial weight shift.

As the baby approaches midline, flex both of the baby's legs (figure 2.3.2), but do not hold the baby's hands. From the position of symmetrical flexion, roll the baby to the other side and repeat the 5-month position with lateral flexion and lower-extremity dissociation.

You must maintain the baby's pelvis in the elevated position and continue to capture the baby's visual attention as you move from side to side with the baby.

Precautions
- Keep the baby's pelvis and leg elevated when in sidelying.
- Maintain the lower leg in extension with continuous traction.
- Keep the lower leg in line with the body.
- Keep the top hip and knee flexed.

Component Goals
- Elongation of the spinal extensors
- Activation of the neck and trunk flexors (abdominals)
- Elongation of the weight-bearing side
- Activation of lateral righting on the nonweight-bearing side
- Activation of neck and trunk flexors with the posterior weight shift from sidelying
- Activation of the neck and trunk extensors with the anterior weight shift from sidelying
- Hip and knee flexion alternating with hip and knee extension
- Lower-extremity dissociation

- Scapulo-humeral mobility
- Sensory feedback of sidelying to facilitate lateral righting reactions
- Sensory awareness of the right and the left sides

Functional Goals

- Lateral righting reactions
- Rolling to sidelying
- Playing in sidelying

2.4 Asymmetrical Sidelying Roll to Prone: 6-Month Roll

This technique is an imitation of how the 6-month-old baby typically rolls from supine to sidelying to prone and back again. This technique can be a continuation of the two previous techniques, the symmetrical 4-month roll, followed by the asymmetrical 5-month roll, followed by the extension of the 6-month roll.

The goal of this facilitation is for the baby to learn to roll from supine to prone. Additional goals include initiation of the movement with antigravity flexion, completion of the movement with antigravity extension, and the transition between flexion and extension made in sidelying with antigravity lateral flexion.

Baby's Position The baby lies supine on the mat.

Therapist's Position Heel-sit in front of the baby in a position to move with the baby (figure 2.4.1). It is important for you to capture the baby's visual gaze with your eyes.

If it is difficult to heel-sit, place the baby on an elevated mat so you can stand during the technique.

Therapist's Hands and Movement

4-Month Roll
Place your index fingers in the baby's palms. Wrap your other fingers around the baby's hands or wrists and hold them securely. Bring the baby's hands toward the baby's knees, place your thumbs under the baby's knees, and flex the baby's knees and hips (figure 2.4.1).

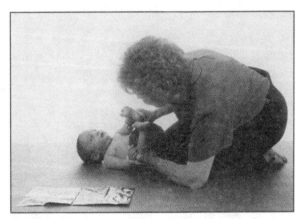

Figure 2.4.1. Asymmetrical sidelying roll to prone: 4-month roll. The therapist places her index fingers in the baby's palms, wrapping her other fingers around the baby's wrists and holding them securely. The therapist brings the baby's hands toward the baby's knees, placing her thumbs under the baby's knees and flexing the baby's knees and hips.

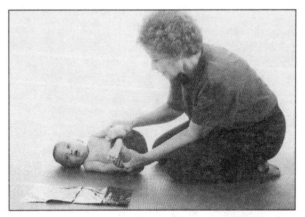

Figure 2.4.2. The therapist holds the baby's flexed legs and rolls the baby symmetrically to the side.

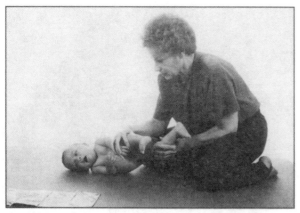 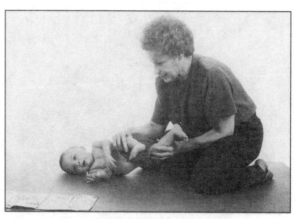

Figure 2.4.3. 5-month roll. The therapist uses her right hand to maintain the top leg in hip and knee flexion and places her top (right) forearm on the baby's pelvis to apply slight pressure from the baby's pelvis diagonally downward to the opposite weight-bearing shoulder. With her left hand, the therapist applies upward traction to the baby's lower hip and knee to extend the hip and knee.

Figure 2.4.4. Backward weight shift. The therapist keeps the baby in sidelying with the legs dissociated and uses her forearm on the baby's pelvis to shift the baby's weight backward to activate the baby's righting reactions, activating the baby's neck and trunk flexors.

While holding the baby's flexed legs, roll the baby symmetrically to the side (figure 2.4.2). Make sure that the baby's head turns with the trunk.

5-Month Roll

Once the baby has rolled to the side, release the baby's bottom hand, maintain the baby's pelvis in the elevated position, place your top forearm on the baby's pelvis, and apply upward traction to the baby's lower hip and knee to extend the hip and knee (figure 2.4.3).

As you lift and extend the baby's lower leg with one hand, maintain the top leg in hip and knee flexion with the other hand (figure 2.4.3). Use the forearm of your top arm to apply slight pressure from the baby's pelvis diagonally downward to the opposite weight-bearing shoulder.

Backward Weight Shift

Keep the baby in sidelying with the legs dissociated, and use your forearm on the baby's pelvis to shift the baby's weight backward, to activate the baby's righting reactions, and thus, activate the baby's neck and trunk flexors (figure 2.4.4).

Note: Compare the baby's face in figures 2.4.3 and figure 2.4.4. As the baby's weight shifts backward in figure 2.4.4, the baby's flexors activate, the baby's head flexes, the mouth closes, and the visual gaze moves downward. Activation of the baby's neck and trunk flexors is important for typical development of the baby's head, mouth, and visual control.

Forward Weight Shift and Completion: 6-Month Roll

From the sidelying position, keep your hands on the baby's legs, and use your forearm on the baby's pelvis to shift the baby's weight forward to activate the baby's righting reactions and thus activate the baby's neck and trunk extensors (figure 2.4.5).

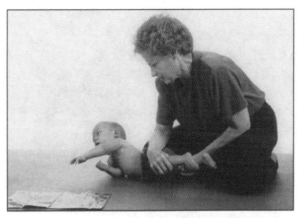

Figure 2.4.5. Forward weight shift and completion: 6-month roll. The therapist uses her forearm on the baby's pelvis to shift the baby's weight forward to activate the baby's righting reactions, activating the baby's neck and trunk extensors.

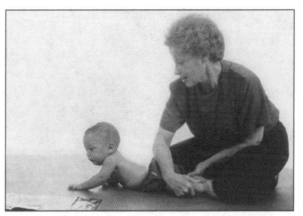

Figure 2.4.6. As the baby approaches prone, the therapist keeps her forearm on the baby's pelvis and applies subtle backward traction to **both** of the baby's legs. The backward movement helps the baby unweight the arm that is under the trunk. The therapist maintains subtle pressure on the baby's pelvis with her forearm.

To complete the baby's transition to prone, maintain your control on the baby's legs and continue to use your forearm on the baby's pelvis to roll the baby's weight forward toward prone (figure 2.4.5).

As the baby approaches prone, keep your forearm on the baby's pelvis and apply subtle backward traction to **both** of the baby's legs (figure 2.4.6). The traction extends the legs and pulls the baby's body backward toward you. The backward movement helps the baby unweight the arm that is under the trunk (figure 2.4.6).

Maintain subtle pressure on the baby's pelvis with your forearm. The downward pressure on the pelvis provides a point of stability and enables the baby to lift the head and upper trunk and bring the arms forward.

Return
To help the baby roll from prone to supine, reverse the procedure.

- Maintain the bottom leg in extension as you flex the top leg at the hip and knee (figure 2.4.5).
- Maintain your forearm on the baby's pelvis and use it to roll the baby to sidelying (figure 2.4.4).
- Once the baby is in sidelying, maintain the top leg in flexion while you flex the bottom leg and bring the baby to supine.

Repeat the roll to the other side. Once you have completed the roll to one side, you do not have to hold the baby's hands to roll to the other side unless the baby uses strong shoulder girdle or humeral retraction.

Suggestion Introduce toys that are interesting to the baby, to motivate the baby to roll and practice goal-directed movement.

Precautions

- Keep the baby's pelvis and leg elevated when in sidelying so the baby will maintain the lateral flexion.
- When completing the transition, maintain the pressure on the baby's pelvis as you apply simultaneous traction to both of the baby's legs.
- Maintain your forearm pressure on the baby's pelvis when the baby is in prone.

Component Goals

- Activation of the neck and trunk flexors
- Elongation of the weight-bearing side
- Hip and knee flexion followed by hip and knee extension
- Lower-extremity dissociation
- Scapulo-humeral mobility
- Forearm weight bearing
- Activation of neck, trunk, and hip extensors
- Sensory feedback of transitioning from supine to prone

Functional Goals

- Independent rolling from supine to prone
- Independent rolling from prone to supine

3. Prone on Lap

3.1   Prone on Lap

The goal of this facilitation is to help the baby tolerate and adjust to the prone position. Additional goals include elongation of the rectus abdominus, hip flexors, and scapulo-humeral muscles; activation of the neck, trunk, and hip extensors; head lifting; and sensory stimulation through the visual, tactile, proprioceptive, and vestibular systems.

The prone position is a very functional position for the baby. From prone the baby can learn to weight shift, dissociate the upper extremities and lower extremities, rise to quadruped, crawl, and rise to stand.

Many babies with developmental delays do not like the prone position because it is difficult for them to rise against gravity. It can be difficult for them to lift their heads in prone and/or to weight bear on their upper extremities. They may not like to weight shift because they lose control and fall over and/or they dislike the varying sensory feedback involved with weight shifts. Obviously there also can be many other reasons. The therapist must evaluate each baby's abilities, dislikes, and impairments to determine why each particular baby dislikes the prone position. The therapist's responsibility then becomes how to help that baby through those impairments so that the baby can become successful.

Baby's Position   The baby lies prone on your lap, with both arms flexed over your leg (figure 3.1.1). This is a good position for babies who have a gastrostomy tube.

Therapist's Position   Long-sit on the floor or sit on a bench or ball, with your hips flexed to 90°. If the baby is long and you must abduct your legs to accommodate the baby's body, check to make sure that the baby's abdomen is not falling between your legs. This will cause the baby's spine to hyperextend. If the baby is too long for your lap, place the baby prone over a bolster or ball.

Therapist's Hands   Place one hand firmly on the baby's hips and pelvis (figure 3.1.1). This provides a stable point from which the baby can lift the head.

You may use your other hand to place a toy in the baby's visual field, or you can place your hand on the baby's trunk to help the baby feel secure. Your hands should be firm but not hard.

If you place both hands on the baby, prearrange the toys so that the baby can look at different heights. If the caregivers attend the session, ask them to hold a toy and move it to different heights.

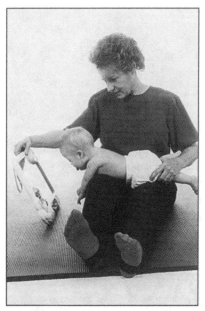

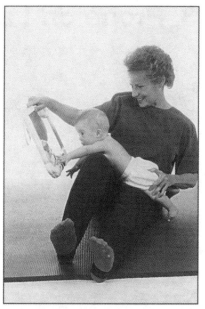

Figure 3.1.1. Prone on lap. The baby lies prone on the therapist's lap with both arms flexed over the therapist's leg. The therapist places one hand firmly on the baby's hips and pelvis.

Figure 3.1.2. The therapist raises her leg to change the baby's prone angle while maintaining the pressure on the baby's hips and pelvis.

Movement There is very little movement involved in this technique.

Raise your leg to change the baby's prone angle (figure 3.1.2). This will increase the baby's visual tracking and upper-extremity reaching. Maintain your pressure on the baby's hips and pelvis.

Some babies have difficulty with the flat prone position. When you elevate your leg, it is easier for the baby to lift the head. When the baby is in a more elevated position, the sensory feedback from the visual and vestibular systems is more comfortable for the baby because it is closer to the feedback in the vertical position.

Suggestions

- Encourage the baby's caregiver to sit in front of the baby and move his or her face to encourage the baby to lift the head.
- Slowly move a toy up and down to encourage head lifting.

Precautions

- Your hands must be firm enough to make the baby feel comfortable and not so hard as to cause discomfort to the baby.
- Move slowly and wait for the baby to lift the head.

Component Goals

- Elongation of rectus abdominus
- Elongation of hip flexors

- Elongation of muscles between the scapula and humerus: teres major, triceps, latissimus dorsi
- Neck, trunk, and hip extension
- Head lifting
- Sensory stimulation through the visual, tactile, proprioceptive, and vestibular systems

Functional Goals

- Preparation for all prone activities
- Ability to adapt and respond to incoming sensory stimulation

3.2 Prone Lateral Weight Shifts

The goal of this facilitation is to increase the baby's tolerance to prone and to lateral weight shifts in prone. Additional goals include elongation of the rectus abdominus, hip flexors, and scapulo-humeral muscles; activation of the neck, trunk, and hip extensors; head lifting and turning from side to side; elongation of the muscles on the weight-bearing side; activation of the neck and trunk muscles for lateral righting; and sensory stimulation through the tactile, proprioceptive, and vestibular systems.

Baby's Position The baby lies prone on your lap, with both arms flexed over your leg.

Therapist's Position Long-sit on the floor, or sit on a bench or ball with your hips flexed to 90°.

Therapist's Hands and Movement: Subtle Weight Shifts For babies who do not tolerate prone very well, and for babies who have difficulty turning the head, your goals will include tolerance to prone and subtle head turning from side to side with the weight shift in the trunk.

Place one hand on the baby's hips and pelvis and the other hand on the baby's rib cage (figure 3.2.1). Spread your fingers to reach around the baby's pelvis and rib cage. Your hands should be firm but not hard.

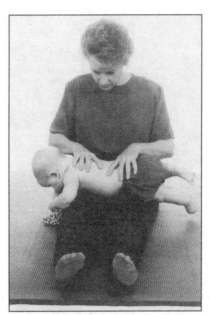 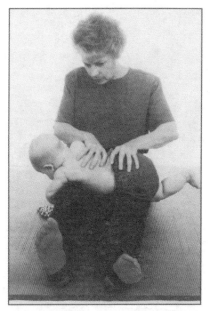 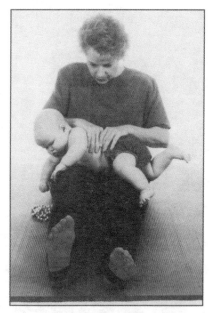

Figure 3.2.1. Prone lateral weight shifts. With the baby lying prone on the therapist's lap with both arms flexed over her leg, the therapist places one hand on the baby's hips and pelvis and the other hand on the baby's rib cage, spreading her fingers to reach around the baby's pelvis and rib cage.

Figure 3.2.2. The therapist slowly shifts the baby's weight to the side, **waiting** for the baby to turn the head.

Figure 3.2.3. As the baby tolerates the weight shifts, the therapist gradually shifts the baby's weight farther to the side until the baby responds with lateral righting of the head and trunk and dissociation of the lower extremities.

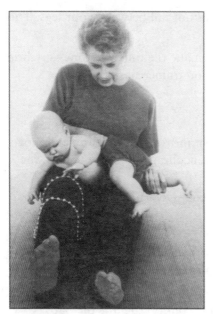

Figure 3.2.4. To increase the baby's elongation on the weight-bearing side, the therapist moves her left hand to the baby's weight-bearing (right) leg, extending the hip and the knee and applying downward traction with slight **internal rotation.** The therapist keeps her right hand on the baby's rib cage to shift the trunk.

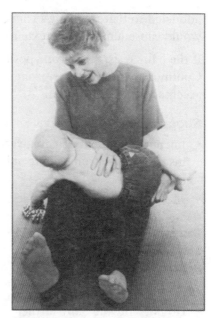

Figure 3.2.5. When shifting the baby's weight away from her, the therapist keeps one hand on the baby's rib cage to shift the baby's trunk, placing her other hand on the baby's weight-bearing leg to extend the hip and the knee and apply downward traction and slight internal rotation.

Slowly shift the baby's weight to the side (figure 3.2.2). Begin with a subtle weight shift and slowly progress to bigger weight shifts. Once you shift the baby's weight to the side, **wait** for the baby to turn the head.

Movement: Larger Weight Shifts When the baby tolerates the weight shifts, gradually shift the baby's weight farther to the side, until the baby responds with lateral righting of the head and trunk and dissociation of the lower extremities (figure 3.2.3).

To increase the baby's elongation on the weight-bearing side, move one of your hands to the baby's weight-bearing leg, extend the hip and the knee, and apply downward traction with slight **internal rotation** (figure 3.2.4). Keep your other hand on the baby's rib cage to shift the trunk. To increase the baby's active participation in the turning, place a toy on your leg where you want the baby to look (figure 3.2.4).

When shifting the baby's weight away from you, keep one hand on the baby's rib cage to shift the baby's trunk. Place your other hand on the baby's weight-bearing leg, extend the hip and the knee, and apply downward traction and slight internal rotation. Use your facial expressions to motivate the baby to turn (figure 3.2.5).

If the baby has difficulty with head lifting, raise one of your legs so that the baby's head is higher than the hips (see figure 3.1.2). Keep your legs adducted so that the baby's trunk does not fall between your legs. This would cause lumbar hyperextension.

If the baby resists the prone position, make the time in prone very brief. Continue to return to the prone position to increase the baby's acceptance of the position.

Suggestions

- Encourage the baby's caregiver to sit in front of the baby and move his or her face from side to side to encourage the baby to turn the head.
- Move a toy from side to side to encourage head turning.

Precautions

- Your hands must be firm enough to make the baby feel comfortable, but not so hard as to cause discomfort to the baby.
- Do not move quickly.
- Do not shift the baby farther than is comfortable for the baby.
- Wait for the baby to turn the head.
- Gradually increase the amount of lateral weight shift.

Component Goals

- Elongation of rectus abdominus
- Elongation of hip flexors
- Elongation of muscles between the scapula and humerus: teres major, triceps, latissimus dorsi
- Head lifting and turning from side to side (head righting)
- Sensory stimulation through the visual, tactile, proprioceptive, and vestibular systems
- Lateral righting of the head and trunk
- Lower-extremity dissociation

Functional Goals

- Preparation for rolling
- Preparation for all lateral weight shifts
- Preparation for the 5-month position
- Ability to adapt and respond to incoming sensory stimulation

3.3 Prone to Sidelying on Lap: Tactile and Visual Body Exploration

The goal of these facilitation techniques is to enable the baby to use tactile and visual feedback to explore body parts, increasing body awareness. Additional goals include facilitation of active reaching and grasping, activation of downward visual gaze, increased tolerance to sidelying, elongation of the muscles on the weight-bearing side, activation of the muscles on the unweighted side toward lateral flexion (lateral head righting and lateral trunk righting), and lower-extremity mobility.

Baby's Position The baby lies in prone on your lap.

Therapist's Position Long-sit on the floor, or sit on a bench or ball with your hips flexed to 90° (figure 3.3.1).

Therapist's Hands and Movement Place one hand on the baby's hips and pelvis and the other hand on the baby's rib cage (figure 3.3.1). Spread your fingers to reach around the baby's pelvis and rib cage. Your hands should be firm but not hard.

Slowly shift the baby's weight to the side until the baby responds with lateral righting of the head and trunk (figure 3.3.2). If the baby tries to retract the unweighted arm, slide your hand around the shoulder and inhibit the retraction (figure 3.3.2). Slide your other hand from the baby's pelvis to the baby's unweighted leg, and flex the leg at the hip and knee (figure 3.3.3). Once you have flexed the baby's leg, slide your hand down to the baby's lower leg and/or foot (figure 3.3.4). You can rest the baby's foot on your leg, but hold it there with your hand.

Note: It is important to slide your hand, rather than lift it to move, so that you can maintain control of the baby's position at all times.

Once the baby is in sidelying, shift the baby's weight slightly posterior to facilitate the flexor muscles (figure 3.3.4). As the baby's flexor muscles become more active, move your hand from the baby's unweighted shoulder to the baby's weight-bearing arm. Use your forearm to support the baby's head.

Bring the baby's hand to the baby's foot (figure 3.3.4) or any part of the leg. Enable or assist the baby to explore the foot and leg with the hand and the eyes.

Use your body to block the baby from rolling backward.

Note: To control the baby's movements, you must position the baby facing away from you. Therefore to repeat these activities on the other side, you must turn the baby around.

Carrying You also can use the sidelying position with lower-extremity dissociation to carry the baby (figure 3.3.5). Place your arm under the baby's weight-bearing arm and hold the baby's flexed leg with your

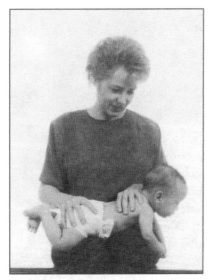

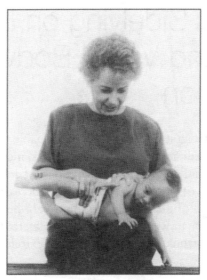

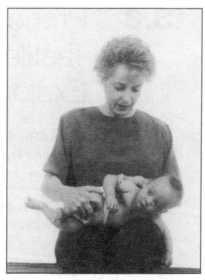

Figure 3.3.1. Prone to sidelying on lap. With the baby lying prone on the therapist's lap, the therapist places one hand on the baby's hips and pelvis and the other hand on the baby's rib cage, spreading her fingers to reach around the baby's pelvis and rib cage.

Figure 3.3.2. The therapist slowly shifts the baby's weight to the side until the baby responds with lateral righting of the head and trunk. The therapist slides her arm around the baby's shoulder to inhibit retraction of the unweighted arm.

Figure 3.3.3. The therapist slides her other hand from the baby's pelvis to the baby's unweighted leg and flexes the leg at the hip and knee.

hand. To control the baby's top arm, place your finger into the baby's hand. Use your other hand to extend and adduct the baby's weight-bearing leg. You also can carry the baby in a more vertical orientation (figure 3.3.6).

Suggestions
- Use an ankle rattle to increase the baby's visual attention and desire to reach to the leg.
- Use hand cream to increase the baby's interest and to vary the baby's tactile input.

Precautions
- Maintain the baby in sidelying by supporting the baby's trunk with your body.
- Keep your forearm under the baby's head.
- Keep the bottom hip and knee extended.
- Keep the top hip and knee flexed.
- Do not move quickly. Give the baby time to respond to and enjoy tactile exploration.

Component Goals
- Lateral weight shifts with lateral righting of the head and trunk
- Elongation of trunk and hip muscles on the weight-bearing side
- Lower-extremity dissociation
- Lower-extremity mobility

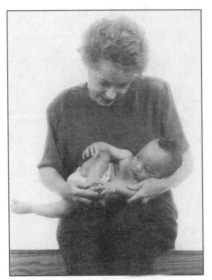

Figure 3.3.4. The therapist shifts the baby's weight slightly posterior to facilitate the flexor muscles. The therapist slides her hand down to the baby's foot and brings the baby's hand to the baby's foot.

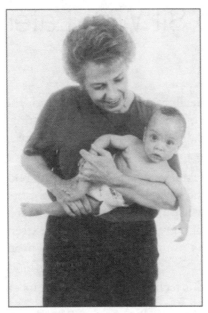

Figure 3.3.5. Carrying. The therapist places her arm under the baby's weight-bearing arm and holds the baby's flexed leg with her hand to carry the baby with lower-extremity dissociation.

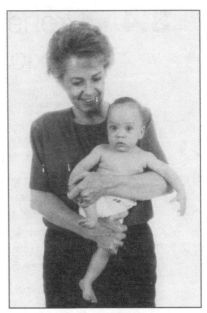

Figure 3.3.6. Carrying the baby in a more vertical orientation. The therapist uses one hand to extend and adduct the baby's weight-bearing leg.

- Upper-extremity reaching
- Visual and tactile exploration of the hand and leg for development of body awareness
- Tactile and proprioceptive input to the weight-bearing foot

Functional Goals
- Increased body awareness
- Directed use of eyes
- Tactile exploration with the hands
- Increased hand use and shaping
- Visual regard of body parts
- Preparation for reaching and playing in sidelying

3.4 Prone to Sit With Lateral Flexion

The goals of these facilitation techniques are for the baby to have the sensory experience of moving from prone to sitting, using lateral flexion to activate the lateral righting reactions, and to prepare for independent transitions to sitting.

Additional goals include movement around the body's axis, elongation of the muscles on the weight-bearing side, activation of the muscles on the unweighted side toward lateral flexion (lateral head righting and lateral trunk righting), preparation for lower-extremity dissociation, and sensory stimulation through the visual, tactile, proprioceptive, and vestibular systems.

You may perform this technique in parts or in its entirety.

Baby's Position The baby lies prone on your lap, with both arms flexed over your leg.

Therapist's Position Long-sit on the floor, or sit on a bench or ball with your hips flexed to 90°.

Therapist's Hands Take your *guiding hand* through the baby's legs and place it on the baby's rib cage (figure 3.4.1). Spread your fingers and thumb so that they span the baby's rib cage and hold it (figure 3.4.1; see also figure 3.4.2). Do not squeeze the baby's rib cage.

Place your *assisting hand* on the baby's arm (figure 3.4.1). Align both of the baby's arms over your leg. Then place your hand on the baby's humerus and shoulder that is close to you (figure 3.4.2).

Movement to Sidelying Use your *guiding hand* on the baby's rib cage to roll the baby to sidelying (figure 3.4.2). As the baby rolls to sidelying, use your *assisting hand* to maintain the baby's bottom arm in shoulder flexion. (You may have to use your forearm to support the baby's head.)

Option: Weight Shifts in Sidelying When the baby is in the sidelying position, use your *guiding hand* on the baby's rib cage to roll the baby backward and forward slowly. Wait for the baby's responses. Rolling the baby backward facilitates the flexors; rolling the baby forward facilitates the extensors. Keep your *assisting hand* on the baby's bottom arm.

Sidelying to Sit From the sidelying position, use your *guiding hand* on the baby's rib cage to shift the baby's weight to the bottom hip as you simultaneously rotate your forearm and bring the baby up to sitting (figure 3.4.3).

Maintain the baby's bottom arm in shoulder flexion with your *assisting hand* and move the baby's bottom arm in synchrony with the trunk as the baby comes up to sit (figure 3.4.3). If the baby needs assistance, use the forearm of your *assisting hand* to support the baby's head during the transition.

Complete the transition all the way to sitting (figure 3.4.4).

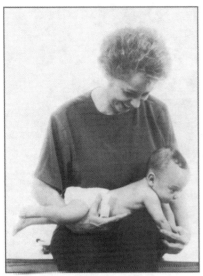

Figure 3.4.1. Prone to sit with lateral flexion. The therapist takes her *guiding hand* through the baby's legs and places it on the baby's rib cage, spreading her fingers and thumb to span and hold the baby's rib cage. The therapist places her *assisting hand* on the baby's arm, aligning both of the baby's arms over her leg.

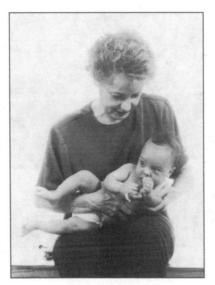

Figure 3.4.2. Movement to sidelying. The therapist places her *assisting hand* on the baby's humerus and shoulder that is closest to her, then uses her *guiding hand* on the baby's rib cage to roll the baby to sidelying. As the baby rolls to sidelying, the *assisting hand* maintains the baby's weight-bearing arm in shoulder flexion.

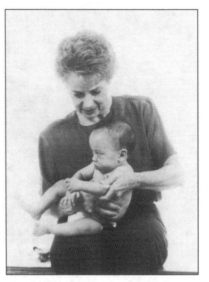

Figure 3.4.3. Sidelying to sit. The therapist uses her *guiding hand* on the baby's rib cage to shift the baby's weight to the bottom hip while simultaneously rotating her forearm and bringing the baby up to sitting. The therapist maintains the baby's bottom arm in shoulder flexion with her *assisting hand* and moves the bottom arm in synchrony with the trunk as the baby comes up to sit.

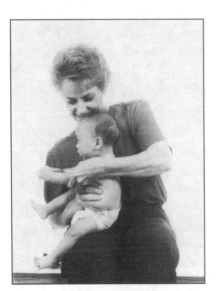

Figure 3.4.4. The therapist completes the transition all the way to sitting.

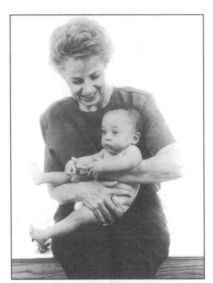

Figure 3.4.5. Sitting to prone. The therapist keeps her arm between the baby's legs and places her *guiding hand* over the baby's lateral hip joint, femur, pelvis, and trunk. The therapist places her assisting-hand arm under the baby's outside arm and reaches for the baby's inside arm.

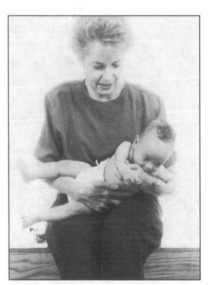

Figure 3.4.6. The therapist applies gentle traction to the baby's arm, bringing it across the baby's chest so that the baby's trunk rotates. The therapist stabilizes the baby's trunk with her *guiding hand*, being careful not to stop the movement and **not to rotate the rib cage over a fixed pelvis.**

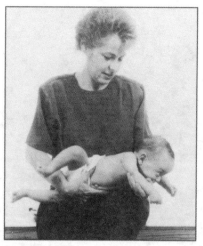

Figure 3.4.7. The therapist continues to support the baby's trunk while continuing to rotate the baby's trunk with traction on the arm.

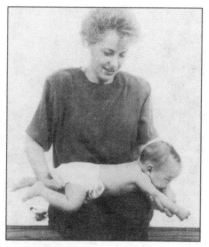

Figure 3.4.8. The therapist carefully lowers the baby's extended body to her legs.

Reverse: Sitting to Prone To return the baby to prone from the sitting position, keep your arm between the baby's legs and place your *guiding hand* over the baby's lateral hip joint, femur, pelvis, and trunk (figure 3.4.5).

Place your *assisting-hand arm* under the baby's outside arm and reach for the baby's inside arm (figure 3.4.5).

Apply gentle traction to the baby's arm and bring it across the baby's chest so that the baby's trunk rotates (figure 3.4.6). Stabilize the baby's trunk with your *guiding hand,* but do not stop the movement (figure 3.4.6). **Do not rotate the rib cage over a fixed pelvis.**

Continue to support the baby's trunk as you rotate it with traction on the arm (figure 3.4.7). Carefully lower the baby's extended body to your legs (figure 3.4.8).

Option: Prone to Sitting Sit on a ball to transition the baby from prone to sitting. It is especially helpful to sit on a ball if the baby responds positively to the proprioceptive and vestibular stimuli provided by bouncing on a ball.

Place one arm between the baby's legs with your *guiding hand* on the baby's trunk, as described in Therapist's Hands on page 56. Start the transition with your *assisting hand* on the baby's arm (figure 3.4.9).

As you transition the baby to sitting, move your *assisting hand* from the baby's arm to the baby's weight-bearing leg (figure 3.4.10). Use your *assisting forearm* to support the baby's trunk and prevent the baby from retracting the shoulder girdle and arm.

Figures 3.4.9 and 3.4.10 illustrate how you must shift your weight when you facilitate the baby's transition from prone to sitting. Your weight shift is especially obvious when you are sitting on a ball, but it also must occur when you are sitting on a bench or the floor.

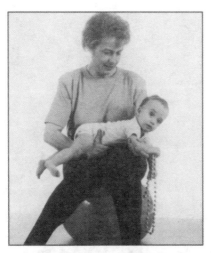 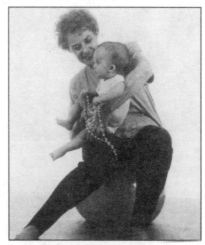

Figure 3.4.9. Prone to sitting. The therapist takes her *guiding hand* through the baby's legs and places it on the baby's rib cage, spreading her fingers and thumb to span and hold the baby's rib cage. The therapist places her *assisting hand* on the baby's arm.

Figure 3.4.10. The therapist transitions the baby to sitting, moving her *assisting hand* from the baby's arm to the baby's weight-bearing leg. The therapist uses the assisting forearm to support the baby's trunk and prevent the baby from retracting the shoulder girdle and arm.

Carrying You also can use the hand placement in this facilitation technique to carry the baby. In figure 3.4.11, the therapist's arm is between the baby's legs with her *guiding hand* on the baby's rib cage. The *assisting-hand arm* supports the baby's trunk as the *assisting hand* holds the baby's leg. (This is similar to figure 3.4.10.)

Figure 3.4.12 is similar to figure 3.4.6.

Precautions

- Do not squeeze the baby's rib cage.
- Keep the baby's weight on the bottom hip. Do not lift the baby into the air with your hand on the baby's trunk.
- Do not move quickly. Move slowly and deliberately to enable the baby to respond to the sensory changes.
- Do not rotate the rib cage over a fixed pelvis.
- If the baby needs head support, keep your forearm under the baby's head.

Component Goals

- Elongation of trunk and hip muscles on the weight-bearing side
- Elongation of muscles between the scapula and humerus: teres major, triceps, latissimus dorsi
- Activation of head, neck, trunk, and hip flexors when rolling backward
- Lateral righting of the head and trunk

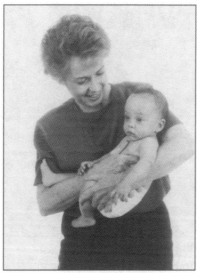 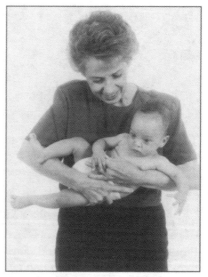

Figure 3.4.11. Carrying. The therapist's arm is between the baby's legs with her *guiding hand* on the baby's rib cage. The assisting-hand arm supports the baby's trunk as her *assisting hand* holds the baby's leg.

Figure 3.4.12. The therapist's *guiding hand* holds the baby's bottom leg in extension and adduction, with her arm supporting the baby's trunk as her *assisting hand* holds the baby's hand.

- Lower-extremity dissociation
- Head, trunk, and hip extension when returning to prone
- Trunk rotation when returning to prone
- Hip rotation as the body pivots on the weight-bearing hip

Functional Goals
- Preparation for head and trunk lateral righting reactions
- Preparation for independent transitions to sitting
- Ability to adapt and respond to incoming sensory stimulation

3.5 Prone to Sit With Extension and Rotation

The goals of this facilitation are for the baby to have the sensory experience of moving from prone to sitting while using extension and rotation and to prepare for independent transitions to sitting. Additional goals include movement around the body's axis, hip and trunk extension with rotation, elongation of the muscles between the scapula and humerus, head rotation and head righting, and sensory stimulation through the visual, tactile, proprioceptive, and vestibular systems.

Baby's Position The baby lies prone on your lap with both arms flexed over your leg.

Therapist's Position Long-sit on the floor (figure 3.5.1), or sit on a bench or ball with your hips flexed to 90°.

Therapist's Hands *Assisting hand:* Place the three middle fingers of one of your hands on the baby's scapula and your thumb and fifth finger around the baby's humerus that is close to you (figure 3.5.1; see the view in figure 3.5.3).

Guiding hand: Place your other hand under the baby's femur that is close to you (near femur). Let the baby's leg rest on your thumb and web space. Place your other fingers on the back of the baby's distant femur (figure 3.5.1).

Movement You can practice the movement in several steps, but it is most effective for the baby when you perform it in its entirety.

Initiate the movement with the thumb on your *guiding hand.* Use your thumb to apply traction to extend and abduct the baby's near femur. (In figures 3.5.1 and 3.5.2, the therapist's left thumb extends and abducts the baby's right femur.) Move your thumb in a clockwise direction. Extend and abduct the hip as far as the baby can tolerate comfortably (figure 3.5.2). As you initiate the movement with the thumb of your *guiding hand,* stabilize the baby's distant femur (the baby's left femur, which is also the weight-bearing femur) with the fingers of your *guiding hand.*

As your *guiding-hand thumb* extends the baby's femur, stabilize the baby's arm and upper trunk with your *assisting hand* (figures 3.5.1 and 3.5.2). This produces trunk rotation with extension.

Once you have rotated the baby's trunk, hold the position with both of your hands and raise your leg that is under the baby's arm (figures 3.5.2 and 3.5.3). As you raise your one leg, shift the baby's weight onto the bottom hip that is resting on your other leg.

As you raise your leg, continue to use your *assisting hand* to stabilize the baby's arm in a forward position, but let the baby's upper trunk move slightly toward rotation with the lower trunk (figure 3.5.3).

As you complete the movement, keep the baby's arm close to the trunk and slide the fingers of your *assisting hand* down the baby's arm (figure 3.5.4).

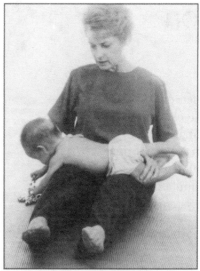

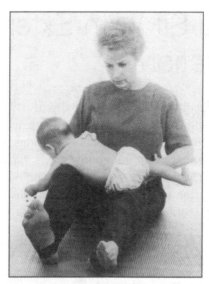

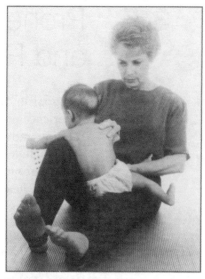

Figure 3.5.1. Prone to sit with extension and rotation. The therapist places the three middle fingers of her right hand on the baby's scapula and the thumb and fifth finger around the baby's right humerus. The therapist places her guiding (left) hand under the baby's right femur, the baby's leg resting on the thumb and web space, with the other fingers of the *guiding hand* on the back of the baby's distant (left) femur. The therapist initiates movement with the thumb of the *guiding hand*, using the thumb to apply traction to extend and abduct the baby's near (left) femur.

Figure 3.5.2. As the guiding-hand thumb extends and abducts the baby's femur as far as the baby can tolerate comfortably, the therapist stabilizes the baby's arm and upper trunk with the *assisting hand*, which produces trunk rotation with extension.

Figure 3.5.3. Once the therapist has rotated the baby's trunk, she holds the position with both hands and raises her leg that is under the baby's arm, shifting the baby's weight onto the bottom hip that is resting on her other leg. The therapist continues to use her *assisting hand* to stabilize the baby's arm in a forward position, letting the baby's upper trunk move slightly toward rotation with the lower trunk.

As the baby comes toward the upright position, use the thumb of your *guiding hand* to place the baby's leg on your leg (figure 3.5.4).

The movement ends with the baby sitting on your lower leg and the baby's arm and trunk resting on your raised leg (figure 3.5.4).

Sitting to Prone
To facilitate the baby from sitting to prone, use the thumb on your *guiding hand* to stabilize the baby's far femur (the baby's right femur in figure 3.5.5). Grasp the baby's nonweight-bearing humerus (right humerus in figure 3.5.5) with your *assisting hand* and adduct the baby's arm to the chest (figure 3.5.4). Apply slight traction to the baby's arm by having the baby reach over your raised leg (figure 3.5.6). Rotate the baby's upper trunk as far as is comfortable for the baby (figure 3.5.6).

When you have rotated the baby's upper trunk as far as it can rotate comfortably, lower your leg, continuing to maintain the baby's leg in abduction and extension but permitting the lower trunk to rotate with the upper trunk (figure 3.5.7). Control the baby's arm and leg until the

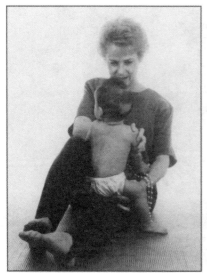

Figure 3.5.4. As the therapist completes the movement, she keeps the baby's arm close to the trunk and slides the fingers of her *assisting hand* down the baby's arm. As the baby comes toward the upright position, the therapist uses the thumb of her *guiding hand* to place the baby's leg on her leg. The movement ends with the baby sitting on the therapist's lower leg and the baby's arm and trunk resting on the therapist's raised leg.

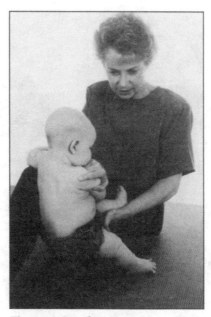

Figure 3.5.5. Sitting to prone. The therapist uses the thumb on her *guiding hand* to stabilize the baby's far (right) femur and grasps the baby's nonweight-bearing (right) humerus with her *assisting hand* to adduct the baby's arm to the chest.

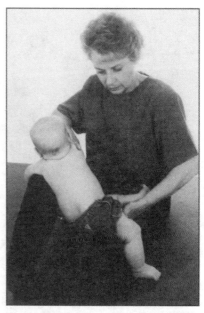

Figure 3.5.6. The therapist applies slight traction to the baby's arm by having the baby reach over her raised leg, then rotates the baby's upper trunk as far as is comfortable for the baby.

baby is prone over your legs. Once the baby is prone, stabilize the baby's hips with your hand (figure 3.5.8).

Precautions

- Do not rotate the baby beyond the baby's comfort level.
- Do not hyperextend the baby's lumbar spine when you extend the baby's leg.
- Do not let the arm retract nor the scapula adduct.
- Do not restrict movement completely in the upper trunk.
- Keep the baby's weight on the bottom hip. Do not lift the baby with your *guiding hand*.
- Do not move quickly.

Component Goals

- Trunk extension with rotation
- Rotation around the body axis
- Hip extension, abduction, and external rotation
- Scapulo-humeral mobility
- Shoulder flexion and horizontal adduction
- Head rotation

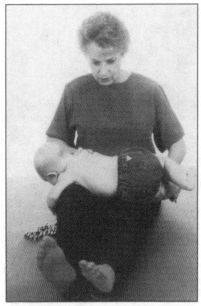 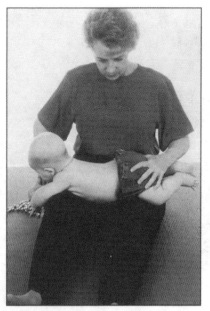

Figure 3.5.7. When the therapist has rotated the baby's upper trunk as far as it can rotate comfortably, the therapist lowers her leg, continuing to maintain the baby's leg in abduction and extension but permitting the lower trunk to rotate with the upper trunk.

Figure 3.5.8. The therapist controls the baby's arm and leg until the baby is prone over her legs, stabilizing the baby's hips with her hand.

Functional Goals

- Preparation for extension with rotation in the trunk for transitional movements
- Preparation for independent transition to sitting
- Controlled sensory stimulation through the visual, vestibular, tactile, and proprioceptive systems
- Preparation for reaching across midline

4. Prone on Ball

4.1 Prone Extension: Forward Weight Shift for Trunk and Hip Extension and Forward Protective Extension

The goals of these facilitation techniques are to increase the baby's trunk and hip extensor range and control; to increase the baby's ability to use the upper extremities in prone activities, upper-extremity weight bearing, and forward protective extension; and to increase the baby's ability to extend the hips and knees for standing and walking.

Baby's Position The baby lies prone over the ball, with the ribs and pelvis well supported by the ball. The baby's arms are in shoulder flexion over the ball (figure 4.1.1).

Therapist's Position Place yourself behind the baby in a position to move forward with the baby.

Therapist's Hands Align the baby's hips in neutral and maintain the hips in extension with your body (figure 4.1.1).

Place your hands on the baby's upper chest and arms (figure 4.1.1). Flex the baby's shoulders with slight external rotation so the baby can reach forward and down to the floor. Maintain this hand placement throughout the movement.

Option Align the baby's hips in neutral and maintain the hips in extension with your forearms (figure 4.1.2).

Place your hands on the baby's arms (figure 4.1.2). Flex the baby's shoulders so the baby can reach forward and down to the floor. Maintain this hand placement throughout the movement.

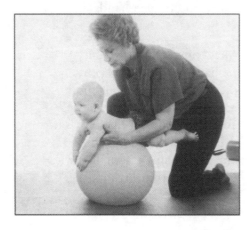

Figure 4.1.1. Prone extension. The baby lies prone over the ball with the ribs and pelvis well supported by the ball, arms in shoulder flexion over the ball. The therapist aligns the baby's hips in neutral and maintains the hips in extension with her body. Placing her hands on the baby's upper chest and arms, the therapist flexes the baby's shoulders with slight external rotation so the baby can reach forward and down to the floor.

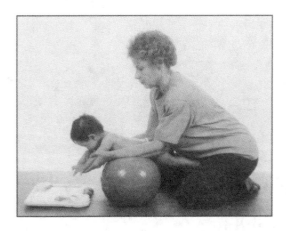

Figure 4.1.2. Option. The therapist places her hands on the baby's arms, flexing the baby's shoulders so the baby can reach forward and down to the floor.

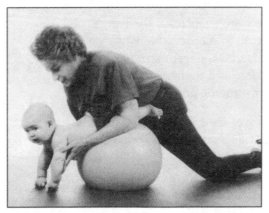

Figure 4.1.3. The therapist guides the baby's weight forward to facilitate upper-extremity forward protective extension while stabilizing the hips and knees in extension and the hips in neutral rotation.

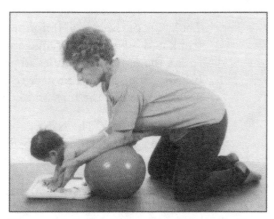

Figure 4.1.4. The baby reaches down to the floor for a toy.

Movement Guide the baby's weight forward to facilitate upper-extremity forward protective extension while stabilizing the hips and knees in extension and the hips in neutral rotation (figures 4.1.3, 4.1.4).

The baby may reach down to the floor for symmetrical protective extension (figure 4.1.3) or to a toy (figure 4.1.4), or the baby may reach straight forward to a wall or mirror to activate the lower trapezius muscles.

If the ball is small, the baby may walk forward on open hands (wheelbarrow).

Optional Hip Control When the baby has some upper-extremity control, you can move your hands to the baby's hips. Place both of your hands on the baby's femurs near the hips and press your thumbs into the baby's gluteus maximus (figure 4.1.5). Bring the baby's hips into neutral alignment with the trunk. Adduct the hips if the baby's legs are abducted, or abduct the hips if the baby's legs are adducted. Depending on the baby's needs, rotate the baby's hips externally or internally to neutral. Maintain this hand placement throughout the movement.

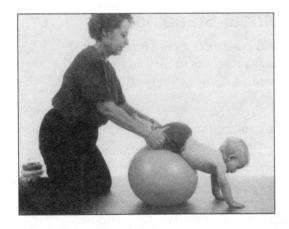

Figure 4.1.5. Optional hip control. The therapist places both hands on the baby's femurs near the hips and presses her thumbs into the baby's gluteus maximus, bringing the baby's hips into neutral alignment with the trunk. The therapist then guides the baby's weight forward to facilitate upper-extremity forward protective extension while stabilizing the hips and knees in extension and the hips in neutral rotation.

Babies who have tight hip flexors or a tight rectus abdominus may try to pull their hips into flexion. The ball helps reduce this pull. Keep the baby in prone but do not force the hips into extension that is beyond the baby's comfort level.

Guide the baby's weight forward to facilitate upper-extremity forward protective extension while stabilizing the hips and knees in extension and the hips in neutral rotation (figure 4.1.5).

Precautions

- Be careful in selecting the size of the ball. The larger the ball, the easier it is for both you and the baby to move. However, the baby will not be able to reach the floor if the ball is too large. Smaller balls enable the baby to reach the hands forward to the floor.
- Always stabilize the baby on the ball.
- Select a speed that is appropriate for the baby, fast enough to stimulate the baby's protective extension response, but not so fast as to frighten the baby.

Component Goals

- Head and trunk extension
- Symmetrical hip and knee extension
- Forward protective extension of the upper extremities
- Upper-extremity weight bearing
- Vestibular and proprioceptive stimulation

Functional Goals

- Preparation of the postural system for extension.
- Forward protective extension of the upper extremities to protect the baby in a fall
- Upper-extremity weight bearing to increase proximal stability (used in transitional movements)

Hip Extension to Symmetrical Standing

Using the same or slightly modified hand placement as in Optional Hip Control, you can bring the baby backward to lower the lower extremities off the ball toward downward protective extension and weight bearing on the feet.

Therapist's Hands Continue to extend and rotate the baby's hips to neutral. Use your hands to press the baby's legs into the ball to secure the baby on the ball. Use your index finger to control the position of the ball.

Keep the thumbs of both hands on and parallel to the femurs. Press up toward the hips. The position and alignment of your thumbs is critical for maintaining the hips in extension. Maintain this hand placement throughout the movement.

Movement While stabilizing the hips and knees in extension and the hips in neutral rotation, guide the baby's weight backward and down toward the floor.

As you bring the baby backward, keep the hips and knees in extension as you place the feet on the floor. It is important to move from weight bearing on the toes to flat-foot weight bearing. The ball assists with trunk extension.

To get the baby's feet flat on the floor, shift the baby's weight posterior and down toward the heels. When the baby's feet are flat on the floor, externally rotate the femurs and tibia to neutral to shift the weight to the lateral borders of the feet.

If the ball is large, you may place the baby's feet initially on your knees. This will help the baby adjust to weight bearing on the feet.

Precautions

- Take care in selecting the size of the ball. If the ball is too large, the baby's feet will not reach the floor. If the ball is too small, it will not support the baby's trunk and the baby may collapse over the ball.
- Maintain control of the ball and the baby on the ball at all times. You may place the ball near a corner to prevent it from rolling away from the baby as the baby comes to standing.
- Maintain lower-extremity alignment in extension and neutral rotation throughout the movement.
- Weight bearing on the balls of the feet stimulates the positive support reaction and can cause the baby to overextend and lose balance. In these cases, the baby should wear neutrally aligned orthotics during lower-extremity weight bearing. Babies who weight bear with excessive pronation also should wear neutrally aligned orthotics.

Component Goals

- Hip and knee extension
- Head and trunk extension

- Lower-extremity weight bearing
- Neutral weight bearing on both feet, that is, weight on the lateral borders of the feet
- Tactile and proprioceptive sensory preparation for the feet to accept weight bearing

Functional Goals

- Preparation of the postural system for extension in standing
- Lower-extremity weight-bearing control for standing and walking
- Weight shift to the lateral borders of the feet, needed in the gait cycle to lock up the foot (loading to terminal stance)

4.2 Upper-Extremity Weight Bearing and Weight Shifts

The goals of these facilitation techniques are to increase the baby's ability to bear weight on the upper extremities and to increase stability in the shoulder girdle muscles for weight-bearing and weight-shifting activities.

Baby's Position The baby lies prone on the ball, with ribs and pelvis well supported by the ball. The baby's arms are in shoulder flexion with the elbows in front of shoulders.

Therapist's Position Kneel behind the baby, and lean your body on the baby's hips to stabilize the baby on the ball.

Forearm Weight Bearing

Therapist's Hands and Movement If the baby's elbows are behind the shoulders (figure 4.2.1), place your hands on the baby's arms, gently move them forward, and adduct them into line with the trunk (figure 4.2.2).

Once the baby's elbows are in front of the shoulders and the baby is bearing weight on the arms, move your hands to the baby's trunk. Reach under the baby's axillae and place your fingers on the baby's pectorals and arms (figure 4.2.3). Press in slightly with the pads of your fingers to activate the pectorals.

Your hands start in a symmetrical position, but you will use them asymmetrically during the weight shifts. The hand on the soon-to-be weight-bearing side is the *guiding hand;* your other hand is the *assisting hand.*

Press slightly on the pectorals with the pads of the fingers of your *guiding hand* and shift the baby's weight laterally. Maintain this pressure to keep the baby's shoulder girdle muscles active (figure 4.2.3). Your *assisting hand* helps with the lateral weight shift and slightly rotates the baby's trunk backward (figure 4.2.3).

If the baby has difficulty maintaining forearm weight bearing, continue with the facilitation to emphasize the weight shifts, trunk rotation, and upper-extremity dissociation (figure 4.2.3).

The weight shift provides sensory stimulation through the visual, vestibular, and somatosensory systems. The weight shift also activates the baby's shoulder girdle muscles for stability on the weight-bearing side and for reaching with the unweighted arm. This prepares the baby for self-initiated weight shifts and reaching.

Practice this technique on each side so each arm has the opportunity to bear weight and each side has the opportunity to reach.

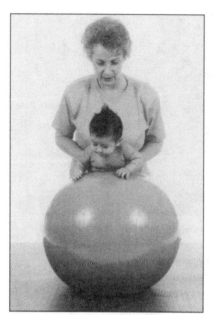

Figure 4.2.1. Forearm weight bearing. The therapist places the baby in prone on the ball with ribs and pelvis well supported by the ball.

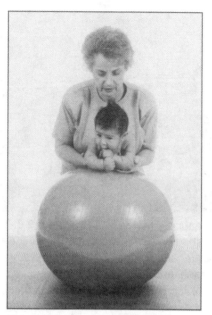

Figure 4.2.2. The therapist places both hands on the baby's arms, gently moving them forward and adducting them into line with the trunk.

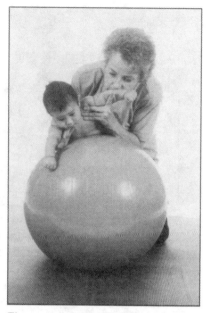

Figure 4.2.3. The therapist moves her hands to the baby's trunk, then reaches under the baby's axillae and places her fingers on the baby's pectorals and arms. The therapist presses slightly on the pectorals with the fingers of the *guiding (right) hand* and shifts the baby's weight laterally, maintaining this pressure to keep the baby's shoulder girdle muscles active. The *assisting (left) hand* helps with the lateral weight shift and slightly rotates the baby's trunk backward.

Extended-Arm Weight Bearing

Therapist's Hands and Movement Bring the baby's arms into shoulder flexion, reach under the baby's axillae, and place your fingers on the baby's pectorals, trunk, and arms (figure 4.2.4). Press in slightly with the pads of your fingers to activate the pectorals. Carefully lean your body on the baby's hips to stabilize the baby on the ball (figure 4.2.4).

Your hands start in a symmetrical position, but you will use them asymmetrically during the weight shifts. The hand on the soon-to-be weight-bearing side is the *guiding hand;* your other hand is the *assisting hand.*

Press slightly on the baby's trunk with the pads of the fingers of your *guiding hand* and shift the baby's weight laterally. Maintain this pressure to keep the baby's shoulder girdle muscles active (figure 4.2.5). You may use your hand on the baby's trunk and your index finger on the baby's arm to stabilize the baby in a weight-bearing position (figure 4.2.5).

Use your *assisting hand* to help with the lateral weight shift, slight trunk rotation, and upper-extremity reaching (figures 4.2.5 and 4.2.6).

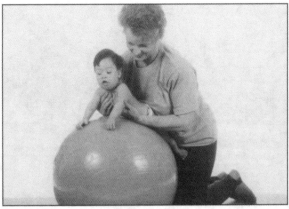

Figure 4.2.4. Extended-arm weight bearing. The therapist brings the baby's arms into shoulder flexion, reaches under the baby's axillae, and places her fingers on the baby's pectorals, trunk, and arms, pressing in slightly with the pads of her fingers to activate the pectorals. The therapist carefully leans her body on the baby's hips to stabilize the baby on the ball.

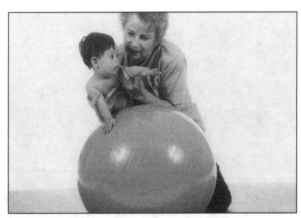

Figure 4.2.5. The therapist presses slightly on the baby's trunk with the pads of the fingers of the *guiding (right) hand* and shifts the baby's weight laterally, using her hand on the baby's trunk and her index finger on the baby's arm to stabilize the baby in a weight-bearing position. The therapist uses the *assisting (left) hand* to help with the lateral weight shift, slight trunk rotation, and upper-extremity reaching.

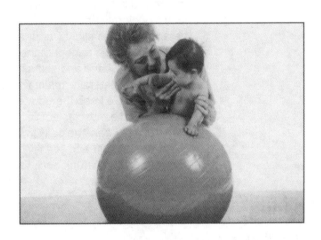

Figure 4.2.6. Option for extended-arm weight bearing. The therapist places her *guiding (left) hand and forearm* on the baby's weight-bearing arm and trunk, stabilizing the baby's trunk with her forearm and hand while using her fingers to externally rotate the baby's arm subtly and press it into the ball. The therapist simultaneously uses her *assisting (right) hand* to rotate the baby's trunk.

Option Place your *guiding hand and forearm* on the baby's weight-bearing arm and trunk (figure 4.2.6). Stabilize the baby's trunk with your forearm and hand while you use your fingers to externally rotate the baby's arm subtly and press it into the ball. Simultaneously use your *assisting hand* to rotate the baby's trunk.

Shift your weight and move into the baby's visual field so the baby can reach for you.

Precautions

- Carefully lean your body on the baby's hips.
- Do not press too strongly into the pectoral muscles.
- Do not elevate the shoulder girdle during the weight shift.
- Control the movement on the weight-bearing side, and keep the weight-bearing side active. (Avoid scapular winging due to an inactive serratus anterior.)

- Rotate the ribs and the pelvis together. Do not rotate the ribs on a fixed pelvis.

Component Goals
- Shoulder girdle control for unilateral weight bearing
- Lateral weight shifts in the upper extremities
- Lateral righting in the head and trunk muscles
- Initiation of cervical and thoracic spine rotational mobility
- Trunk extension with rotation
- Elongation of the rectus abdominus
- Hip extension with elongation of the hip flexors

Functional Goals
- Lateral righting of the head and trunk for transitional movements
- Upper-extremity weight bearing and weight shifting control for upper-extremity dissociation (right-left) needed for crawling and climbing
- Face-side upper-extremity reaching enabling eye-hand regard during reaching
- Increased reaching and grasping skills on the unweighted side

4.3 Lateral Righting Reactions and Sideways Protective Extension

The goals of this facilitation are to increase the baby's lateral righting reactions of the head and trunk and sideward protective extension reactions of the upper and lower extremities. You also can work on upper-extremity weight bearing and pushing.

Baby's Position The baby lies prone over the ball, with ribs and pelvis well supported by the ball. The baby's arms are in shoulder flexion over the ball.

Therapist's Position Kneel beside the ball.

Therapist's Hands and Movement

Weight Shift Away From You
Hold the baby's arm and leg that are away from you (figure 4.3.1). Place one of your hands proximally on the baby's arm near the shoulder and your other hand on the baby's leg near the hip. Use both of your hands to stabilize the baby on the ball. Be aware that you must be able to support and control the baby during the weight shift and that you may have to modify your hand placement to do so.

While holding the baby's arm and leg securely, roll the ball **slightly** away from you. As you roll the ball, apply slight traction to both the baby's arm and leg. This will shift the baby's weight away from you (figure 4.3.2). The baby should respond to the lateral weight shift with lateral righting of the head and trunk back toward you, reaching with the unweighted arm, and flexion of the hip and knee on the unweighted leg (figure 4.3.3).

You can assist the baby's lateral response by bringing your face into the baby's visual field, tipping the ball farther, and/or moving the ball at varied speeds while maintaining the baby's stability on the ball.

Return to Midline
Keep the same hand placement and return the baby to midline. Stabilize the baby in midline and slowly move your hands, one at a time, to the baby's opposite arm and leg.

Weight Shift Toward You
With the baby returned to midline, slowly move your hands, one at a time, and hold the baby's arm and leg that are closest to you (figure 4.3.4). Place one hand proximally on the arm near the shoulder and the other hand on the leg near the knee.

Roll the ball slightly toward you. At the same time, apply traction to the baby's arm to flex the baby's shoulder and to the baby's leg to extend the baby's hip and knee (figure 4.3.5). Simultaneous traction to the arm and leg elongates the baby's side and helps shift the baby's weight to that side (figure 4.3.5).

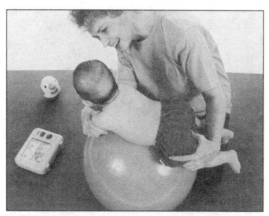

Figure 4.3.1. Lateral righting reactions and sideways protective extension: Weight shift away from therapist. The therapist holds the baby's arm and leg that are away from her, placing her right hand proximally on the baby's arm near the shoulder and her left hand on the baby's leg near the hip, then using both hands to stabilize the baby on the ball.

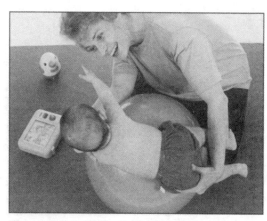

Figure 4.3.2. While holding the baby's arm and leg securely, the therapist rolls the ball slightly away from her, applying slight traction to both the baby's arm and leg, which shifts the baby's weight away from her.

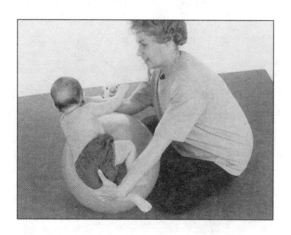

Figure 4.3.3. The baby responds to the lateral weight shift with lateral righting of the head and trunk back toward the therapist, reaching with the unweighted arm, and flexing of the hip and knee on the unweighted leg.

Use both hands to stabilize the baby on the ball. You must be able to support and control the baby during the weight shift and may have to modify your hand placement to do so.

Options

- If the baby can accept the position and does not have low tone or ligamentous laxity, maintain your hands on the baby's arm and leg that are close to you, roll the ball away from you, and bring the baby's top arm and leg closer together (figure 4.3.6). Approximation of the baby's arm and leg help the baby laterally flex the head and trunk. **If the baby has low tone and ligamentous laxity, this is not an appropriate technique.**

  Bring the baby's weight back toward you by applying traction and separating the baby's arm and leg (figure 4.3.5).

- If the baby has sufficient control for lateral flexion and does not have low tone or ligamentous laxity, continue to approximate the baby's arm and leg and to roll the ball away from you until the baby

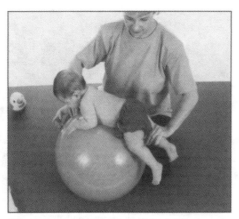

Figure 4.3.4. Weight shift toward therapist. The therapist stabilizes the baby in midline, then slowly moves her hands, one at a time, to the baby's opposite arm and leg.

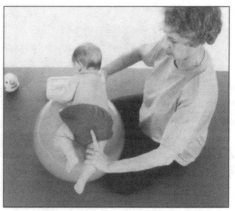

Figure 4.3.5. The therapist holds the baby's arm and leg closest to her, placing one hand proximally on the arm near the shoulder and the other hand on the leg near the knee. The therapist then rolls the ball slightly toward her, at the same time applying traction to the baby's arm to flex the baby's shoulder and to the baby's leg to extend the baby's hip and knee.

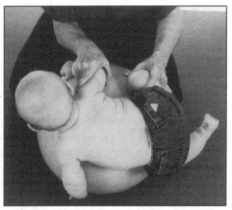

Figure 4.3.6. Option for lateral flexion of head and trunk. The therapist keeps her hands on the baby's arm and leg that are close to her, then moves the ball away and brings the baby's top arm and leg closer together. The therapist shifts the baby's weight back toward her as in figure 4.3.5.

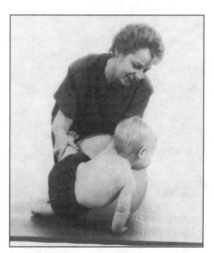

Figure 4.3.7. Option for abduction and protective extension of bottom arm and leg. The therapist continues to approximate the baby's arm and leg and to roll the ball away from her until the baby responds with abduction and protective extension of the bottom arm and leg.

responds with abduction and protective extension of the bottom arm and possibly the bottom leg (figure 4.3.7). If the baby puts weight onto the bottom arm, encourage the baby to push with that arm. **If the baby has low tone and ligamentous laxity, this is not an appropriate technique.**

Bring the baby's weight back toward you by applying traction to and separating the baby's arm and leg (figure 4.3.5).

Precautions

- Be careful when holding the baby's extremities and shifting the weight. Use a smooth and continuous, not a jerky, weight shift. A jerky movement may put too much stress on the joints.
- You must be able to control the baby during the whole range of the weight shifts. Therefore, you should move only in the range where you can maintain control of the baby.
- You must grade the speed of the movement and allow the baby time to respond. Some babies respond best to faster movement. Other babies need more time to respond. If the movement is too fast, the baby may hold on to the ball and not respond with other reactions. Some babies are too trusting and feel no need to respond. For these babies, it is often necessary to wait for a response in a shifted position.
- **Do not use** the optional hand placement for weight shifts away from you if the baby has low tone or ligamentous laxity.

Component Goals

- Lateral righting of the head and trunk
- Elongation of the weight-bearing side
- Abduction and protective extension of the free extremities

Functional Goals

- Stimulation to the vestibular and visual systems to help them learn to respond with lateral righting during lateral weight shifts
- Sideward protective extension of the limbs, to protect the baby in case of a fall

4.4 Prone to Sit on the Ball

The goals of this facilitation are to increase the baby's trunk and hip mobility into extension and rotation and to teach the baby a strategy to transition from prone to sitting.

Baby's Position The baby lies prone over the ball, with the trunk and pelvis well supported by the ball. The baby's arms are in shoulder flexion over the ball, and the hips are extended (figure 4.4.1).

Therapist's Position Kneel beside the baby.

Therapist's Hands *Assisting hand:* Place the index and middle fingers of your *assisting hand* on the baby's shoulder and your thumb and fifth finger around the baby's humerus that is close to you (figure 4.4.1; see views in figures 4.4.2 and 4.4.3).

Guiding hand: Place your *guiding hand* under the baby's femur that is close to you, with your fingers on the baby's distant femur (figure 4.4.1). Place the thumb of your *guiding hand* on the baby's femur that

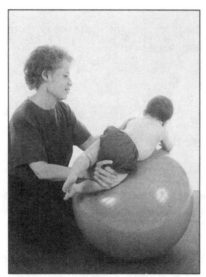

Figure 4.4.1. Prone to sit on the ball. The baby lies prone over the ball. The therapist places the index and middle fingers of her *assisting hand* on the baby's shoulder and her thumb and fifth finger around the baby's humerus that is close to her. She places her *guiding hand* under the baby's femur that is close to her, with her fingers on the baby's distant femur and her thumb on the baby's femur that is close to her, using that thumb to apply traction to extend and abduct the baby's near hip.

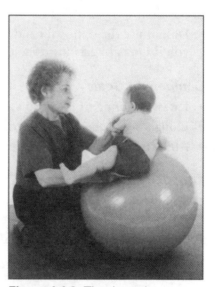

Figure 4.4.2. The therapist continues to stabilize the baby's arm in the forward position with her *assisting hand* and extends and abducts the baby's leg as far as is comfortable.

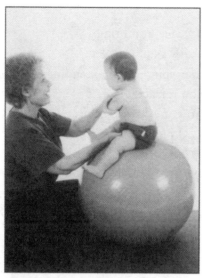
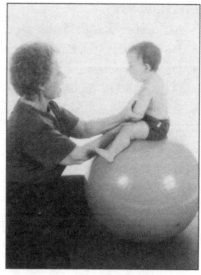

Figure 4.4.3. When the therapist has extended and abducted the baby's leg as far as is comfortable, the therapist uses her *assisting hand* to bring the baby to sitting, simultaneously using the thumb on her *guiding hand* to lower the baby's femur onto the ball.

Figure 4.4.4. The therapist completes the transition to sitting by using her thumb to rotate the baby's femur externally to shift the baby's weight to symmetrical sitting.

is close to you (figures 4.4.1 and 4.4.3). Your thumb will facilitate most of the movement.

Movement Stabilize the baby's arm and upper trunk in the forward position with your *assisting hand*. Use the thumb of your *guiding hand* to apply traction to extend and abduct the baby's near hip (figure 4.4.1). Extend and abduct the hip as far as the baby can tolerate comfortably.

Continue to stabilize the baby's arm in the forward position with your *assisting hand*, but when you have extended and abducted the baby's leg as far as is comfortable, use your *assisting hand* to bring the baby to sitting (figures 4.4.2 and 4.4.3). Simultaneously use the thumb on your *guiding hand* to lower the baby's femur onto the ball (figure 4.4.3).

Complete the transition to sitting by using your thumb to rotate the baby's femur externally to shift the baby's weight to symmetrical sitting (figure 4.4.4). Note how the baby's left leg has moved from internal rotation in figure 4.4.3 toward external rotation in figure 4.4.4. External rotation of the baby's left femur shifts the baby's weight to the left.

Stabilize the baby's arm close to the trunk throughout the transition.

Throughout the movement, as you shift the baby's weight away from you, subtly move the ball toward you. This ensures that the baby's hips remain on the ball and that the baby does not roll off the ball.

It is important to perform this transition on each side to ensure symmetry in the trunk and in the upper and lower extremities.

Precautions

- Make sure that the baby is safe and stable at all times.
- Do not rotate the baby beyond the baby's comfort level.
- Do not hyperextend the baby's lumbar spine when extending the hip.
- Do not let the baby's arm close to you retract.
- Do not let the baby's scapula close to you adduct.
- Stabilize the baby's arm in the forward position but do not restrict movement completely in the upper trunk.
- Keep the baby's weight on the bottom hip. Do not lift the baby with your *guiding hand*.
- When moving the baby on the ball, it is important to keep the baby's pelvis and hip on the ball, which means that you must move the ball subtly under the baby.
- Do not move quickly.

Component Goals

- Rotation around the body axis
- Trunk extension with rotation
- Hip extension, abduction, and external rotation on the unweighted/moving leg
- Shoulder flexion and horizontal adduction
- Head rotation

Functional Goals

- Preparation for extension with rotation in the trunk for transitional movements
- Preparation for independent transition to sitting
- Increased rib cage and intercostal mobility to increase respiration
- Controlled sensory stimulation to improve postural adjustments and control

5. Prone on Floor

5.1   Shoulder Girdle Facilitation for Lateral Weight Shifts

The goal of this facilitation is to activate the baby's shoulder girdle muscles so that the baby can sustain shoulder girdle control during prone weight shifting to reach and play with one hand and subsequently to use reciprocal arm movements to crawl.

Baby's Position   The baby lies prone or in forearm weight bearing on the floor with the hips extended.

Therapist's Position   Kneel behind the baby.

Therapist's Hands and Movement   Flex the baby's shoulders so that the baby's elbows are in front of the baby's shoulders. Place your hand under the baby's axilla with your fingers on the baby's pectorals and your thumb on the baby's humerus along the triceps (figure 5.1.1). Use your other hand to hold and move the toy.

Use the pads of your fingers to press slightly on the baby's pectorals and rib cage to activate the baby's pectorals and serratus anterior to bring the baby to forearm weight bearing (figure 5.1.1). Once the baby's shoulder girdle muscles are active and the scapula actively abducts, use your fingers to shift the baby's weight laterally. Apply slight traction to the baby's arm with your thumb. The traction helps the baby to elongate the side.

As the baby's weight shifts to one arm, the baby's opposite arm is free to reach. Use a toy that is interesting to the baby to facilitate the reach (figures 5.1.2 and 5.1.3).

Facilitate the weight shift and the reaching to each side (figure 5.1.3).

Suggestion   To motivate the baby to participate actively in the activity and to "practice" the activity, use toys that are interesting to the baby. Toys that have cause-effect properties and are easy to activate with one hand are most appropriate.

Precautions
- Your hand must maintain the activation of the pectorals and serratus anterior without pressing with force.
- Give the baby time to respond to the weight shift and reach for the toy.

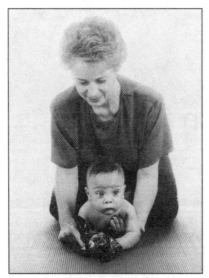

Figure 5.1.1. Shoulder girdle facilitation for lateral weight shifts. The therapist places her left hand under the baby's axilla with her fingers on the baby's pectorals and her thumb on the baby's humerus along the triceps. She uses the pads of her fingers to press slightly on the baby's pectorals and rib cage to activate the baby's pectorals and serratus anterior to bring the baby to forearm weight bearing. Once the baby's shoulder girdle muscles are active and the scapula actively abducts, the therapist uses her fingers to shift the baby's weight laterally and applies slight traction to the baby's arm with her thumb.

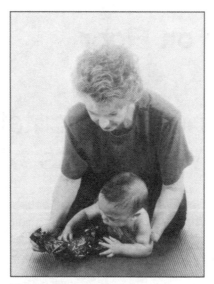

Figure 5.1.2. To facilitate the reach, the therapist uses her other hand to hold and move a toy that is interesting to the baby.

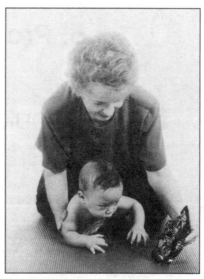

Figure 5.1.3. The therapist facilitates the weight shift and the reaching to the baby's other side.

Component Goals
- Shoulder girdle stability for unilateral weight shifts
- Reaching with the face-side hand
- Head and trunk lateral righting
- Elongation on the weight-bearing side

Functional Goals
- Forearm weight shifting in floor play
- Face-side reaching for toys in floor play
- Preparation for creeping, crawling, and climbing

5.2 Sidelying: Play in Sidelying

The goal of this facilitation is to activate the baby's shoulder girdle muscles so the baby can sustain shoulder girdle control during prone weight shifting and sidelying. Additional goals include reaching and playing with one hand, elongation of the weight-bearing side, lateral flexion of the head and trunk, and lower-extremity dissociation.

Baby's Position The baby lies prone or in forearm weight bearing on the floor with the hips extended.

Therapist's Position Kneel beside the baby.

Therapist's Hands and Movement Place your *guiding hand* under the baby's axilla with your fingers on the lateral portion of the baby's pectorals and your thumb on the baby's humerus along the triceps (see figure 5.2.3, therapist's right hand).

Place your *assisting hand* on the lateral-anterior portion of the baby's rib cage, not on the pelvis, to maintain the alignment between the ribs and pelvis (figure 5.2.1, therapist's left hand). This hand **assists** with the lateral weight shift **only if** the baby has difficulty. It is important not to pull the baby with this hand.

Use the pads of the fingers of your *guiding hand* to press slightly on the baby's pectorals and rib cage to activate the baby's pectorals and serratus anterior to bring the baby to forearm weight bearing (figure 5.2.1). Once the baby's shoulder girdle muscles are active, use your fingers to shift the baby's weight laterally (figure 5.2.2). Apply slight traction to the baby's weight-bearing arm with your thumb. The traction helps the baby to elongate the side with eccentric muscle activity.

If the baby needs more help rolling to sidelying, use your *assisting hand* to guide the baby's rib cage to sidelying (figure 5.2.2).

As the baby's weight shifts to one arm, the baby's other arm is free to reach. Use a toy that is interesting to the baby to facilitate the reach (figures 5.2.2 and 5.2.3).

As the baby rolls to sidelying, the unweighted side laterally flexes and the lower extremities dissociate. The weighted/bottom leg extends, adducts, and internally rotates to neutral; the unweighted/top leg flexes, abducts, and externally rotates (figure 5.2.2). The bottom leg must remain extended at the hip and knee to keep the trunk active. If the bottom leg flexes, the trunk will become inactive.

Once the baby is in sidelying, move your *assisting hand* to the baby's unweighted/top leg and flex the baby's hip and knee so the baby's foot can rest on the mat (figure 5.2.3). The baby can continue to play with the toy in this position (figure 5.2.3).

Remove the toy if you want to encourage the baby to play with the hand on the foot (figure 5.2.4). Hand-on-foot play helps the baby learn about body parts and helps the baby to learn to use the hands. It also decreases tactile sensitivity of the hand and foot.

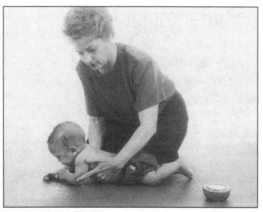

Figure 5.2.1. Play in sidelying. The therapist places her *guiding (right) hand* under the baby's axilla with her fingers on the lateral portion of the baby's pectorals and her thumb on the baby's humerus along the triceps, using the pads of the fingers of the *guiding hand* to press slightly on the baby's pectorals and rib cage to activate the baby's pectorals and serratus anterior and bring the baby to forearm weight bearing. The therapist places her *assisting hand* on the lateral-anterior portion of the baby's rib cage, not on the pelvis, to maintain the alignment between the ribs and pelvis.

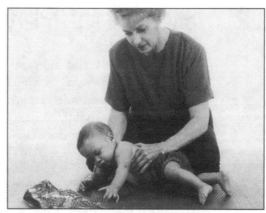

Figure 5.2.2. The therapist uses her *guiding hand* fingers to shift the baby's weight laterally, applying slight traction to the baby's weight-bearing arm with her thumb. The traction helps the baby to elongate the side with eccentric muscle activity. The therapist uses her *assisting hand* to guide the baby's rib cage to sidelying. As the baby rolls to sidelying, the unweighted side laterally flexes and the lower extremities dissociate. The weighted/bottom leg extends, adducts, and internally rotates to neutral; the unweighted/top leg flexes, abducts, and externally rotates.

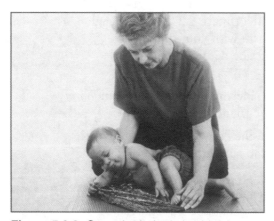

Figure 5.2.3. Once the baby is in sidelying, the therapist moves her *assisting hand* to the baby's unweighted/top leg and flexes the baby's hip and knee so the baby's foot can rest on the mat.

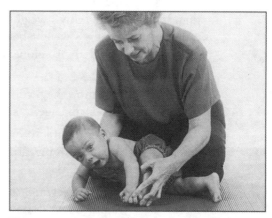

Figure 5.2.4. The therapist removes the toy to encourage the baby to play with the hand on the foot. She uses her index finger to hold the baby's hand on the foot.

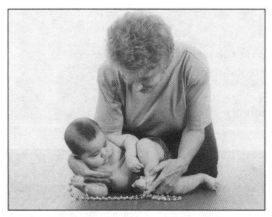

Figure 5.2.5. Option: For the baby who cannot maintain forearm weight bearing and/or cannot laterally flex the head, the therapist places her *guiding hand* under the baby's head and guides it toward lateral flexion, supporting the baby's head as she presents a toy and the baby's foot for the baby to explore.

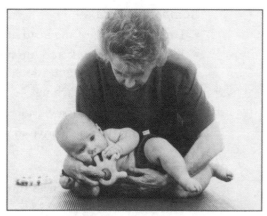

Figure 5.2.6. Option: For the baby who has difficulty with lower-extremity dissociation, the therapist places her *assisting hand* between the baby's legs and onto the baby's trunk, supporting the baby's head with her *guiding hand* and presenting a toy for the baby to explore.

Note: For you to control the baby's movements, the baby must face away from you. Therefore, to repeat these activities on the other side, you must turn the baby so that the baby is facing the other direction, that is, to the right instead of the left.

Options If the baby cannot maintain forearm weight bearing and/or cannot laterally flex the head, place your *guiding hand* under the baby's head and guide it toward lateral flexion (figures 5.2.5 and 5.2.6).

- Support the baby's head as you present toys and/or the baby's foot for the baby to play with, explore visually and tactually (figure 5.2.5), or explore in the mouth (figure 5.2.6).
- If the baby has difficulty with lower-extremity dissociation, place your *assisting hand* between the baby's legs and onto the baby's trunk (figure 5.2.6). Use your forearm to flex the top leg.

Precautions
- Maintain the baby in well-aligned sidelying.
- Keep your hand on the baby's pectorals and keep the baby's pectorals active.
- If the baby cannot laterally flex the head, place and keep your hand or forearm under the baby's head.
- Keep the bottom hip and knee extended.
- Keep the top hip and knee flexed.
- Do not move quickly. Give the baby time to respond to tactile exploration.
- Move deliberately and enable the baby to initiate and lead the play.

Component Goals

- Lateral righting of the head and trunk
- Elongation of trunk and hip muscles on the weight-bearing side, especially the latissimus dorsi and hip abductors
- Upper-extremity reaching
- Lower-extremity dissociation and mobility
- Tactile and proprioceptive input to the weight-bearing foot

Functional Goals

- Increased body awareness through visual and tactile exploration
- Directed use of eyes
- Tactile exploration with the hands
- Increased functional hand use for play
- Visual regard of body parts
- Preparation for reaching and playing in sidelying

5.3 Prone to Sitting

The goal of this facilitation is for the baby to learn to transition from prone to sitting. Additional goals include sensory stimulation with adaptation to the changing environment as the baby moves around the body axis, spinal mobility, facilitation of lateral righting reactions with activation of the muscles that laterally flex the head and trunk, upper-extremity weight bearing and pushing, and lower-extremity dissociation.

Baby's Position The baby lies prone or in forearm weight bearing on the floor with the hips extended.

Therapist's Position Kneel beside the baby.

Therapist's Hands and Movement Place your *guiding hand* under the baby's arms and flex both of the baby's shoulders so that the baby's arms are in front of the baby (figure 5.3.1). Use your *assisting hand* to extend the baby's hips (figure 5.3.1).

Once you have flexed the baby's shoulders, slide your *guiding hand* to the baby's lateral rib cage and pectorals, then place your *assisting hand* on the baby's lateral rib cage farthest away from you (figure 5.3.2).

Use your *assisting hand* to extend the baby's hips (figure 5.3.1), then place your *assisting hand* on the baby's lateral rib cage farthest away from you (figure 5.3.2).

Activate the baby's pectorals by pressing in slightly with the pads of the fingers of your *guiding hand*. When the baby's pectorals become active, rotate the baby's trunk to shift the baby's weight toward you (figure 5.3.2). Then slightly lift the baby's trunk while shifting the baby's weight to the bottom hip (figure 5.3.2).

Use your *assisting hand* to **help** rotate the baby's rib cage. **Do not pull the baby up with this hand**. Move slowly and give the baby time to prop on the extended arm (figure 5.3.2). You want the baby to learn to push up actively to sitting so that this becomes a functional movement.

As the baby rises, continue to rotate the baby's trunk (rib cage and pelvis) over the bottom hip (figure 5.3.3). Simultaneously use both of your hands to press the baby's trunk subtly toward the bottom hip. Do not rotate the rib cage over the pelvis.

Transition the baby to full upright symmetrical sitting (figure 5.3.4). Maintain your hands on the baby's trunk while giving symmetrical downward pressure into the base of support.

You can use the same hand placement to reverse the baby's movement and facilitate the baby back to prone.

Precautions
- The *guiding hand* must maintain the activation of the pectorals without pressing with force.
- The *assisting hand* must not pull the baby to sitting.

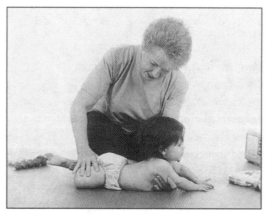

Figure 5.3.1. Prone to sitting. The therapist places her *guiding hand* under the baby's arms and flexes both of the baby's shoulders so that the baby's arms are in front of the baby. The therapist uses her *assisting hand* to extend the baby's hips.

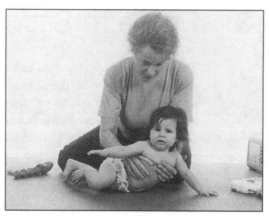

Figure 5.3.2. The therapist slides her *guiding hand* to the baby's lateral rib cage and pectorals, then places her *assisting hand* on the baby's lateral rib cage farthest away from her. The therapist activates the baby's pectorals by pressing in slightly with the fingers of her *guiding hand*. As the baby's pectorals become active, the therapist rotates the baby's trunk to shift the baby's weight toward her, then slightly lifts the baby's trunk while shifting the baby's weight to the bottom hip, moving slowly to give the baby time to prop on the extended arm.

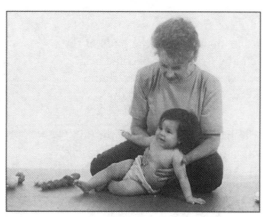

Figure 5.3.3. As the baby rises, the therapist continues to rotate the baby's trunk (rib cage and pelvis) over the bottom hip, simultaneously using both hands to press the baby's trunk subtly toward the bottom hip without rotating the rib cage over the pelvis.

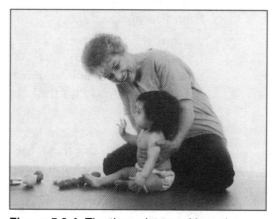

Figure 5.3.4. The therapist transitions the baby to full, upright, symmetrical sitting, maintaining her hands on the baby's trunk while giving symmetrical downward pressure into the base of support.

- Do not place your *assisting hand* on the pelvis.
- Do not stop in side-sitting. Continue up to symmetrical sitting. You want the baby to learn to sit symmetrically and to move into and out of symmetry. If you stop in side-sitting, the baby may have difficulty learning to sit with symmetry. Also, side-sitting is not a preferred position because the baby can rotate the rib cage over a stable pelvis when side-sitting, which leads to abnormal dissociation of the rib cage and pelvis.

Component Goals

- Movement around the body axis
- Trunk rotation
- Upper-extremity weight bearing and weight shifting
- Pelvic-femoral (hip joint) mobility
- Somatosensory input into the base of support for subsequent postural preparations and reactions in sitting

Functional Goals

- Independent transition from prone to sitting
- Independent transition from sitting to prone
- Preparation for upper-extremity lateral protective extension reactions in sitting

5.4 Prone to Runner's Stretch Position

The goals of this facilitation are to activate the shoulder girdle and trunk muscles for extended-arm weight bearing with elbow extension and trunk extension, to dissociate the lower extremities, and to increase mobility in both lower extremities.

Baby's Position The baby lies prone or in forearm weight bearing on the mat with the hips extended.

Therapist's Position Kneel beside the baby.

Therapist's Hands and Movement Reach your *guiding hand* under the baby's axilla and place it on the baby's lateral rib cage and pectorals. Use your *assisting hand* to extend the baby's hips (figure 5.4.1).

Activate the baby's shoulder girdle muscles by pressing in slightly on the pectorals with the pads of the fingers of your *guiding hand*. Simultaneously facilitate a lateral weight shift by using an arc-like movement with your hand (wrist flexion) (figure 5.4.2). Maintain the activation of the shoulder girdle muscles with your *guiding hand*, and place your *assisting hand* on the unweighted leg, bringing the hip and knee into maximum flexion (figure 5.4.2).

Once you have flexed the hip and knee, slide your *assisting hand* backward so that you can hold the baby's leg in flexion and stabilize the baby's pelvis simultaneously. Continue to use your *guiding hand* on the baby's pectorals to activate the shoulder girdle and lift the baby's trunk over and onto the flexed leg (figure 5.4.3).

When the baby's weight is on the flexed leg, place your *assisting hand* across the baby's sacrum (figure 5.4.4) and press the pelvis downward and backward to maintain the dissociated position of the legs. It is especially important to maintain the downward and backward pressure; otherwise the baby will try to move to quadruped, especially if the hip flexors are tight.

Continue to use your *guiding hand* on the baby's pectorals to activate the shoulder girdle.

Once the pelvis and trunk are over the flexed leg, you can facilitate weight shifts from side to side. Continue to use your *assisting hand* to maintain your backward control on the baby's sacrum, and use your *assisting hand* to shift the baby's weight from side to side. Make sure that the ankle on the baby's flexed leg is plantarflexed (figure 5.4.4). The baby should respond with lateral righting of the head and trunk on the unweighted side and elongation of the muscles on the weighted side when the weight shifts from side to side.

Runner's Stretch to Extended-Leg Quadruped
From the runner's stretch position, you can facilitate the baby into a modified quadruped position and maintain the lower-extremity dissociation (figure 5.4.5).

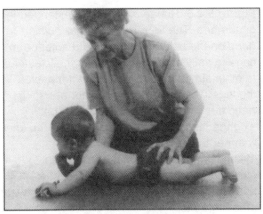

Figure 5.4.1. Prone to runner's stretch position. With the baby in forearm weight bearing on the mat with the hips extended, the therapist reaches her *guiding hand* under the baby's axilla and places it on the baby's lateral rib cage and pectorals, using the *assisting hand* to extend the baby's hips.

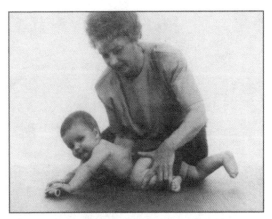

Figure 5.4.2. The therapist activates the baby's shoulder girdle muscles by pressing in slightly on the pectorals with the pads of the *guiding-hand fingers*, simultaneously facilitating a lateral weight shift by using an arc-like movement with the hand (wrist flexion). The therapist places her *assisting hand* on the unweighted leg and brings the hip and knee into maximum flexion.

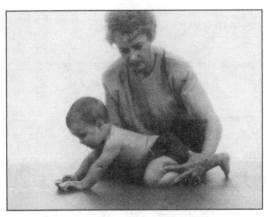

Figure 5.4.3. The therapist slides her *assisting hand* backward to hold the baby's leg in flexion and stabilize the baby's pelvis simultaneously. She continues to use her *guiding hand* on the baby's pectorals to activate the shoulder girdle and lift the baby's trunk over and onto the flexed leg.

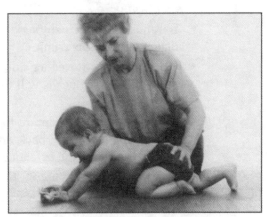

Figure 5.4.4. With the baby's weight on the flexed leg, the therapist places her *assisting hand* across the baby's sacrum and presses the pelvis downward and backward to maintain the dissociated position of the legs.

Use your *guiding hand* on the baby's pectorals and anterior rib cage to activate the baby's trunk muscles and to maintain the baby's weight posteriorly on the legs.

Move your *assisting hand* from the baby's sacrum to the baby's extended leg. Grasp the leg near the knee with your thumb parallel to the femur. Maintain the baby's hip and knee in extension, carefully lift the baby's leg, and shift the baby's weight forward onto the arms (figure 5.4.5).

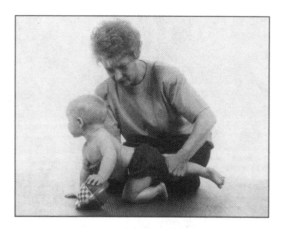

Figure 5.4.5. Runner's stretch to extended-leg quadruped. The therapist uses her *guiding hand* on the baby's pectorals and anterior rib cage to activate the baby's trunk muscles and to maintain the baby's weight posteriorly on the legs. The therapist moves her *assisting hand* from the baby's sacrum to the baby's extended leg and grasps the leg near the knee with her thumb parallel to the femur. Maintaining the baby's hip and knee in extension, the therapist carefully lifts the baby's leg and shifts the baby's weight forward onto the arms.

You can use the baby's leg to move back and forth from runner's stretch to quadruped and to shift the baby's weight laterally. Internally rotate and lower the leg to facilitate the baby's weight to shift toward the extended-leg side; externally rotate and slightly lift the leg to shift the baby's weight toward the flexed-leg side. Maintain your *guiding hand* on the baby's trunk at all times to keep the pectoral and abdominal muscles active throughout the transitions.

Precautions

- You must keep the baby's extended leg extended and in neutral alignment with the trunk.
- Keep the baby's flexed leg adducted under the trunk. If you enable the leg to abduct, the pelvis will tilt anteriorly and the lumbar spine will hyperextend.
- The easiest way to maintain lower-extremity dissociation is to keep the pressure down and back on the pelvis. If you reduce the pressure, the baby will flex the extended leg and assume a quadruped position.
- Never force the baby into a position that is uncomfortable for the baby.

Component Goals

- Head lifting and righting on the sagittal plane
- Upper-extremity, extended-arm weight bearing
- Elongation of the trunk muscles on the weight-bearing side
- Lateral flexion of the spine and lateral righting of the head, trunk, and pelvis on the unweighted side
- Lower-extremity dissociation, including increased range of motion at the hips and knees (elongation of the hip and knee flexors on the extended leg, elongation of the hip and knee extensors on the flexed leg, and elongation of the hip abductors and adductors on both legs).
- The marked lower-extremity dissociation prevents the pelvis from moving on the sagittal plane, thus preventing it from moving into an anterior or posterior pelvic tilt. Therefore, the movements around the pelvis and lumbar spine occur on the frontal and transverse plane.

Functional Goals

- Lateral righting of the head and trunk, basic postural reactions, and actions the baby uses to maintain postural control and balance
- Lower-extremity dissociation, essential to all transitional movements such as crawling, climbing, and walking
- Transitions from prone to quadruped

5.5 Prone Straddle

The goals of this facilitation are to increase the baby's trunk and hip extensor control and weight bearing and weight shifting on the upper extremities for crawling and climbing.

Baby's Position The baby is prone with both legs extended, abducted, and resting on your flexed legs (figure 5.5.1).

Therapist's Position Kneel-sit with the baby's legs resting on your legs.

Therapist's Hands Place your hands on the lateral sides of the baby's trunk, with your index fingers or thumbs on the baby's arms to stabilize the arms (figures 5.5.1 and 5.5.3). Place your forearms laterally on the baby's legs to stabilize them on your flexed legs (figure 5.5.1).

Keep both hands on the baby's trunk during the facilitation.

Movement While stabilizing the baby's hips and knees in extension and the hips in neutral rotation, press lightly on the baby's pectorals with your fingers to activate the baby's shoulder girdle muscles (figure 5.5.1). Once you have activated the shoulder girdle muscles, rotate the baby's trunk so the baby's weight shifts laterally onto one arm (figures 5.5.2 and 5.5.3).

This enables the baby to reach with the unweighted hand. Shift the weight to each side so each arm has the experience of weight shifting, weight bearing, and reaching.

Suggestion Use a toy that is appropriate for the baby to engage with while in the weight-bearing position.

Precaution The baby's shoulder girdle and abdominal muscles must be active during the entire activity. If they are not active, you will observe a lumbar lordosis or an anterior pelvic tilt.

Component Goals
- Head and trunk extension
- Head and trunk rotation
- Hip and knee extension
- Upper-extremity weight bearing
- Upper-extremity lateral weight shifts
- Radial-ulnar weight shifts in the hands
- Elongation of the wrist and finger flexors

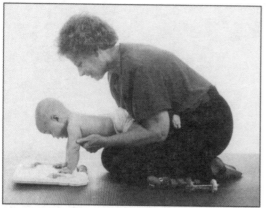

Figure 5.5.1. Prone straddle. The baby is prone with both legs extended, abducted, and resting on the therapist's flexed legs. The therapist places her hands on the lateral sides of the baby's trunk, with thumbs on the baby's arms to stabilize the arms and forearms placed laterally on the baby's legs to stabilize them on the therapist's flexed legs. While stabilizing the baby's hips and knees in extension and the hips in neutral rotation, the therapist presses lightly on the baby's pectorals with her fingers to activate the baby's shoulder girdle muscles.

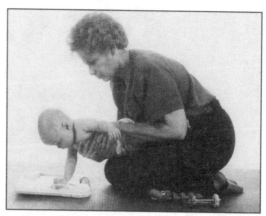

Figure 5.5.2. The therapist rotates the baby's trunk so the baby's weight shifts laterally onto one arm.

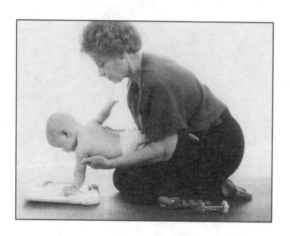

Figure 5.5.3. The therapist shifts the baby's weight to the other side so the other arm has the experience of weight shifting, weight bearing, and reaching.

Functional Goals

- Preparation of the postural system for extension
- Upper-extremity weight bearing and weight shifting to increase the dynamic proximal stability at the shoulder girdle. The baby will use this stability in transitional movements and to retrieve toys or objects that are out of the immediate range.
- Preparation for development of the arches of the hands

6. Prone on Bolster

6.1   Sitting to Prone on Bolster: Symmetrical Hip Extension

The goal of this facilitation is for the baby to learn to transition from sitting to prone on the bolster. Additional goals include shoulder flexion, trunk rotation, and rotation around the body axis.

Baby's Position   The baby sits beside the bolster (figure 6.1.1).

Therapist's Position   Kneel or heel-sit behind the baby.

Therapist's Hands and Movement   Place both of your hands on the baby's trunk and extend the baby's trunk (figure 6.1.1). Use both hands to rotate the baby's trunk. As the baby rotates toward the bolster, slide your hands from the baby's trunk to the baby's arms (figure 6.1.2), and place the baby's arms over the bolster.

Keep your hands on the baby's arms, stabilize the baby's trunk with your forearms, and roll the baby onto the bolster.

Once the baby's trunk is well supported on the bolster, move your hands to the baby's hips (figure 6.1.3). Place both hands on the baby's femurs near the knees, with your thumbs parallel to the baby's femurs. Externally rotate the femurs to neutral and extend the hips and knees into line with the pelvis and trunk (figure 6.1.3).

Options

- Stabilize the baby in the extended position and encourage the baby to use the hands to play (see figure 6.2.1).
- While stabilizing the baby's hips in extension and neutral rotation, quickly, but carefully, guide the baby's weight forward over the bolster at various speeds to elicit a **forward protective extension** reaction (figure 6.1.4). Move the baby forward far enough so the baby's hands make contact with the surface. Do not move the baby quickly if the baby has limited ability to respond.

Precautions

- Keep the baby's hips in neutral rotation to ensure activation of the gluteus maximus. If the legs internally rotate, the gluteus maximus does not work and the lumbar spine hyperextends.
- Keep the baby's pelvis on the bolster so the lumbar spine does not hyperextend.
- Watch the baby's hand placement to make sure that the weight remains on the palmar surface.

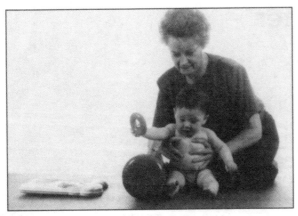

Figure 6.1.1. Sitting to prone on bolster: Symmetrical hip extension. The therapist places both hands on the baby's trunk and extends the baby's trunk, then uses both hands to rotate the baby's trunk.

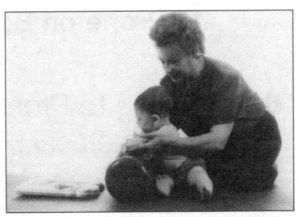

Figure 6.1.2. As the baby rotates toward the bolster, the therapist slides her hands from the baby's trunk to the baby's arms. Stabilizing the baby's trunk with her forearms, the therapist places the baby's arms over the bolster, then rolls the baby onto the bolster.

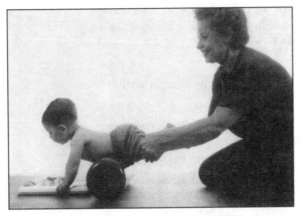

Figure 6.1.3. Once the baby's trunk is well supported on the bolster, the therapist moves her hands to the baby's hips, placing both hands on the baby's femurs near the knees, thumbs parallel to the baby's femurs. The therapist externally rotates the femurs to neutral and extends the hips and knees into line with the pelvis and trunk.

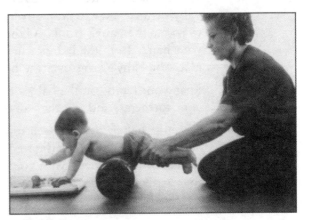

Figure 6.1.4. Option to elicit forward protective extension. While stabilizing the baby's hips in extension and neutral rotation, the therapist quickly, but carefully, guides the baby's weight forward over the bolster at various speeds to elicit a forward protective extension reaction, moving the baby forward far enough so the baby's hands make contact with the surface.

- If you try to facilitate **forward protective extension,** make sure that the baby has some ability to respond. If the baby has limited ability to respond, perform this technique on a ball, which will provide more support to the baby.

Component Goals
- Trunk rotation with symmetrical shoulder flexion
- Hip extension with activation of the gluteus maximus
- Symmetrical trunk extension
- Upper-extremity weight bearing and weight shifting for increased proprioception and stability

- Active shoulder flexion with elbow, wrist, and finger extension
- Elongation of wrist and finger flexors

Functional Goals

- Increased control of trunk and hip extensors to use in upright postures
- Forward protective extension to prevent injury when falling forward
- Preparation of the arms for extended-arm weight bearing to use for crawling and climbing
- Elongation of wrist and finger flexors for increased use of hands
- Finger-palm dissociation when the weight is on the heel of the hands and the fingers are free to flex/extend and rake

6.2 Prone to Sidelying With Lower-Extremity Dissociation

The goals of this facilitation are to increase the baby's trunk mobility and control and to increase the baby's lower-extremity mobility, dissociation, and active muscle control.

Baby's Position The baby lies prone over the bolster, with the trunk well supported by the bolster. The baby's arms are in shoulder flexion over the bolster. The baby's trunk, pelvis, and hips are horizontal and in neutral alignment with each other (figure 6.2.1).

Therapist's Position Kneel-sit behind the baby.

Therapist's Hands and Movement Place your hands on the lateral sides of the baby's femurs over the knees, with your thumbs on and parallel to the femurs (figures 6.2.1, 6.2.2). Extend the baby's hips and knees and align them to neutral. Extend the baby's legs as far as is comfortable for the baby. If the baby fights the position, do not resist the baby.

Your *guiding hand* is on the baby's soon-to-be bottom leg. Most of the control of this facilitation technique comes from the facilitation of the bottom leg. Your *assisting hand* is on the soon-to-be top leg.

To dissociate the baby's lower extremities, apply backward traction to one of the baby's legs with your *guiding hand* while you internally rotate the leg to neutral (figure 6.2.2, right leg). You must perform the traction and the internal rotation simultaneously. Keep the hip and knee in extension, parallel to and in line with the trunk. Maintain the baby's hip extension with your thumb (see figure 6.2.4).

Simultaneous traction with internal rotation of the lower extremity results in elongation of the baby's entire side (shoulder girdle to pelvic girdle) and causes the baby's weight to shift to that side. (The bottom side is the elongated side.)

As you shift the baby's weight to one side, slide your *assisting hand* to the knee and tibia of the baby's other leg and guide the leg into flexion, abduction, and external rotation (figures 6.2.2 and 6.2.3). As you flex the leg, approximate the femur into the pelvis to roll the baby backward (figure 6.2.3).

When the baby's weight shifts and the bottom side elongates, the baby responds with lateral righting or lateral flexion on the topside (figure 6.2.3). Contraction of the abdominals and flexion, abduction, and external rotation of the unweighted lower extremity accompanies lateral righting of the head, trunk, and pelvis.

It is helpful to place or move toys into the baby's visual field to stimulate the baby to participate with and complete the movement (figure 6.2.3).

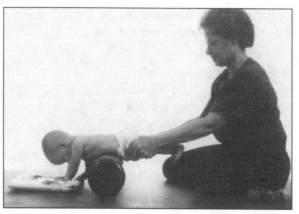

Figure 6.2.1. Prone to sidelying with lower-extremity dissociation. The baby lies prone over the bolster, with the trunk well supported by the bolster. The baby's arms are in shoulder flexion over the bolster. The baby's trunk, pelvis, and hips are horizontal and in neutral alignment with each other. The therapist places her hands on the lateral side of the baby's femurs over the knees, her thumbs on and parallel to the femurs.

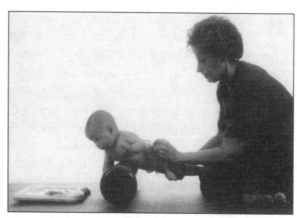

Figure 6.2.2. To dissociate the baby's lower extremities, the therapist applies backward traction to the baby's right leg with her *guiding hand*, at the same time rotating the leg internally to neutral. As the baby's weight shifts to one side, the therapist slides her *assisting hand* to the knee and tibia of the baby's left leg, guiding the leg into flexion, abduction, and external rotation.

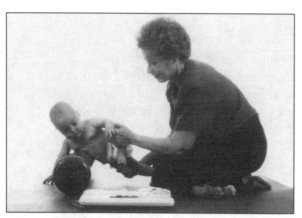

Figure 6.2.3. As the therapist flexes the left leg with her *assisting hand*, she approximates the femur into the pelvis to roll the baby backward.

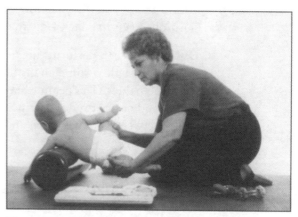

Figure 6.2.4. The therapist facilitates the weight shift to the other side, maintaining the baby's hip extension with the *guiding-hand thumb*.

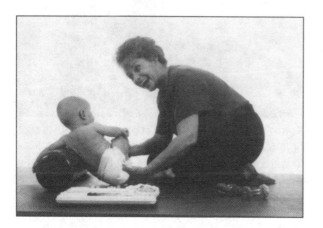

Figure 6.2.5. To increase the elongation of the baby's weight-bearing side, the therapist slowly lowers the baby's hip to the floor with her *guiding hand* while maintaining the baby's legs in dissociation, using her *assisting hand* to press the baby's flexed femur into the pelvis so the pelvis rotates slightly backward.

To return the baby to symmetry, roll the baby's weight forward on the bolster, extend and internally rotate the baby's flexed leg to neutral, and maintain the extended leg in extension.

From symmetry, facilitate the weight shift to the other side (figure 6.2.4). To increase the elongation of the baby's weight-bearing side, slowly lower the baby's hip to the floor with your *guiding hand* while maintaining the baby's legs in dissociation (figure 6.2.5). Use your *assisting hand* to press the baby's flexed femur into the pelvis so the pelvis rotates slightly backward. This keeps the baby's abdominals active. Make sure that the baby's arm stays on the bolster.

Sidelying to Foot Placement

To increase the baby's lower-extremity dissociation and hip and trunk extension, facilitate the baby into the sidelying position with lower-extremity dissociation, and lower the baby's body toward the floor (figure 6.2.6). Place the foot of the baby's flexed leg on the floor with your *assisting hand* while keeping the back leg extended with your *guiding hand* (figure 6.2.6).

As you place the baby's foot on the floor, shift the baby's weight slightly forward onto the bolster (figure 6.2.7). Once the baby's foot is in a weight-bearing position, press down through the knee to the foot with your *assisting hand* to help the baby maintain the weight-bearing position. Keep the back leg extended.

Option You can perform this technique on a peanut ball (figure 6.2.8). The peanut ball is softer than the bolster and thus is more comfortable for some babies. The peanut may be easier for you to use because it is bigger and easier to move than the bolster, and the baby rests in the valley between the two ends, and thus, is more secure.

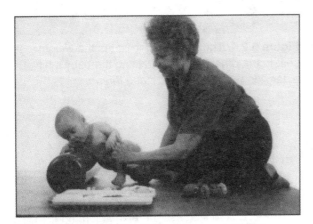

Figure 6.2.6. Sidelying to foot placement. The therapist facilitates the baby into the sidelying position with lower-extremity dissociation, then lowers the baby's body toward the floor. The therapist places the foot of the baby's flexed leg on the floor with her *assisting hand*, keeping the back leg extended with her *guiding hand*.

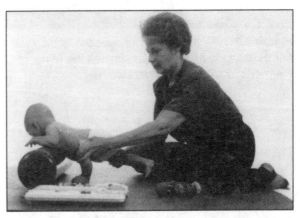

Figure 6.2.7. As the therapist places the baby's foot on the floor, she shifts the baby's weight slightly forward onto the bolster. Once the baby's foot is in a weight-bearing position, the therapist presses down through the knee to the foot with her *assisting hand* to help the baby maintain the weight-bearing position, keeping the back leg extended with her *guiding hand*.

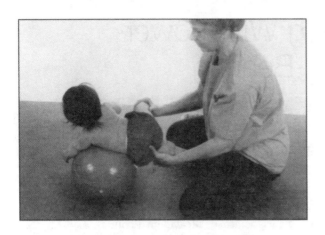

Figure 6.2.8. Option: The therapist performs the Prone to Sidelying With Lower-Extremity Dissociation facilitation on a peanut ball.

Precautions

- Keep the baby's bottom leg in extension and in line with the trunk in order to keep the trunk active. **If the bottom leg flexes, the trunk becomes inactive.**
- What you do with your *guiding hand* is what controls the baby's movements. Pay close attention to the traction of the leg with extension and internal rotation.
- Do not be aggressive with your *assisting hand*. Use it to assist the baby's initiation of hip flexion, abduction, and external rotation of the unweighted leg.
- Gently approximate the baby's flexed femur into the pelvis to rotate the baby's trunk slightly backward. The backward movement of the trunk activates the baby's abdominal muscles.

Component Goals

- Elongation of the muscles on the weight-bearing side: scapulo-humeral muscles, intercostals, muscles between the ribs and pelvis (especially the oblique abdominals, latissimus dorsi, and quadratus lumborum), and the pelvic femoral muscles (hip abductors, adductors, flexors, and extensors)
- Active lateral flexion, lateral righting of the head, trunk (spine), and pelvis on the unweighted side
- Activation of the abdominal muscles with a backward weight shift
- Lower-extremity dissociation and increased range of motion at the hips and knees

Functional Goals

- Lateral righting of the head and trunk are basic postural reactions used to maintain balance and initiate transitions.
- All transitional movements such as reciprocal crawling, climbing, and walking use lower-extremity dissociation.

6.3 Prone to Sidelying With Lower-Extremity Weight-Bearing Progression

The goals of these facilitation techniques are to increase the baby's trunk mobility and control and to increase the baby's lower-extremity mobility, dissociation, and active muscle control.

These techniques are a continuation of the previous technique, 6.2, Prone to Sidelying With Lower-Extremity Dissociation. However, Prone to Sidelying With Lower-Extremity Weight-Bearing Progression emphasizes lower-extremity dissociation, mobility, weight bearing, and transitions that use lateral weight shifts.

Baby's Position The baby lies prone over the bolster, with the trunk well supported by the bolster. The baby's arms are in shoulder flexion over the bolster. The baby's trunk, pelvis, and hips are horizontal and in neutral alignment with each other (figure 6.3.1).

Therapist's Position Kneel-sit behind the baby.

Therapist's Hands and Movement Place your hands on the lateral side of the baby's femurs over the knees, with your thumbs on and parallel to the femurs (figure 6.3.1). Extend the baby's hips and knees and align them to neutral. Extend the baby's legs as far as is comfortable for the baby. If the baby fights the position, do not resist the baby.

Your *guiding hand* is on the baby's soon-to-be-bottom, weight-bearing leg. Most of the control of this facilitation technique comes from the facilitation of the bottom leg. Your *assisting hand* is on the soon-to-be-flexed top leg.

To dissociate the baby's lower extremities, apply backward traction to one of the baby's legs with your *guiding hand* while you rotate the leg internally to neutral (figure 6.3.2, right leg). You must perform the traction and the internal rotation simultaneously. Keep the hip and knee in extension, parallel to and in line with the trunk. Maintain the baby's hip extension with your thumb (see figure 6.2.4).

As you shift the baby's weight to one side, slide your *assisting hand* to the knee and tibia of the baby's other leg and guide the leg into flexion, abduction, and external rotation (figure 6.3.2). As you flex the leg, approximate the femur into the pelvis to roll the baby backward (figure 6.3.2) and activate the abdominal muscles.

Sidelying to Elongated Side-Sit and Foot Placement

Once you have dissociated the baby's legs (figure 6.3.2), keep the bottom hip and knee in extension and lower the extended leg to the

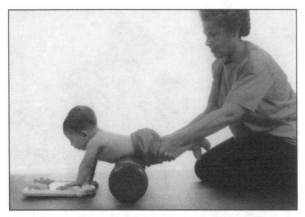

Figure 6.3.1. Prone to sidelying. The baby lies prone over the bolster with the trunk well supported by the bolster. The baby's arms are in shoulder flexion over the bolster. The baby's trunk, pelvis, and hips are horizontal and in neutral alignment with each other. The therapist places her hands on the lateral side of the baby's femurs over the knees, thumbs on and parallel to the femurs, extending the baby's hips and knees and aligning them to neutral.

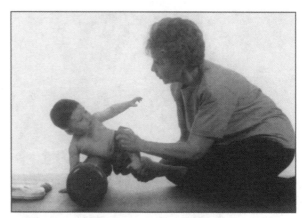

Figure 6.3.2. To dissociate the baby's lower extremities, the therapist applies backward traction to the baby's right leg with her *guiding hand*, at the same time rotating the leg internally to neutral. As the baby's weight shifts to one side, the therapist slides the *assisting hand* to the knee and tibia of the baby's left leg, guiding the leg into flexion, abduction, and external rotation and approximating the femur into the pelvis to roll the baby backward and activate the abdominal muscles.

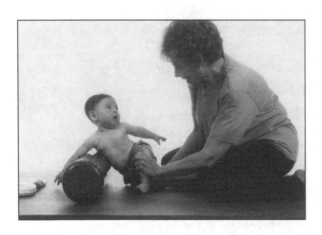

Figure 6.3.3. Sidelying to elongated side-sit and foot placement. The therapist keeps the bottom hip and knee in extension and lowers the extended leg to the floor with her *guiding hand*. The therapist keeps the top leg flexed at the hip and knee, aligning the tibia perpendicular to the floor and placing the baby's foot on the floor with her *assisting hand*.

floor (figure 6.3.3) with your *guiding hand*. **Extension of the hip on this side is necessary to keep the trunk active.** If hip flexion occurs, the weight-bearing side of the trunk will become inactive and sag.

Keep the top leg flexed at the hip and knee, align the tibia perpendicular to the floor, and place the baby's foot on the floor with your *assisting hand* (figure 6.3.3).

Once the foot is in a weight-bearing position, press down through the baby's knee to the foot with your *assisting hand* to help the baby maintain the weight-bearing position.

When the baby's foot is in a weight-bearing position, use your *assisting hand* to approximate the femur into the pelvis and shift the baby's trunk backward. Apply traction to the femur to shift the trunk forward.

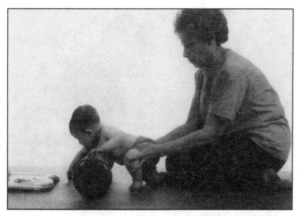

Figure 6.3.4. Elongated side-sit to half-kneel. The therapist shifts the baby's weight slightly forward onto the bolster, keeping her *guiding hand* on the extended leg and guiding it into hip and knee flexion, then stabilizing the hip and pressing the knee into the floor. The therapist uses her *assisting hand* to stabilize the flexed leg in a weight-bearing position, spreading her fingers to stabilize the baby's femur and tibia.

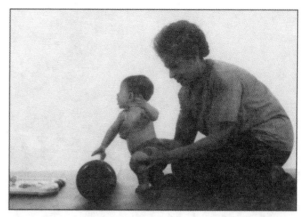

Figure 6.3.5. The therapist maintains her *assisting hand* on the baby's forward leg and carefully moves her *guiding hand* from the baby's hip to the baby's trunk, lifting the baby's trunk so the back hip extends and the baby assumes a half-kneel position.

The backward and forward weight shifts increase the baby's pelvic-femoral mobility, elongate the hamstrings, and increase ankle joint mobility.

Elongated Side-Sit to Half-Kneel

Once the baby is in the elongated side-sit position with the bottom leg extended and the top leg flexed with the foot stabilized on the floor, shift the baby's weight slightly forward onto the bolster (figure 6.3.4). **Keep your hands on both of the baby's legs.**

As the baby's weight shifts forward, keep your *guiding hand* on the extended leg and guide it into hip and knee flexion (figure 6.3.4). As the hip flexes, use your *guiding hand* to stabilize the hip and press the knee into the floor.

Use your *assisting hand* to stabilize the flexed leg in a weight-bearing position. You may have to spread your fingers to stabilize the baby's femur and tibia (figure 6.3.4).

When the baby's lower extremities and pelvis are stable, maintain your *assisting hand* on the baby's forward leg and carefully move your *guiding hand* from the baby's hip to the baby's trunk (figure 6.3.5). If the baby's hips remain stable in the dissociated position, lift the baby's trunk so the back hip extends and the baby assumes a half-kneel position (figure 6.3.5).

The baby may bear weight on the upper extremities and push up with the arms.

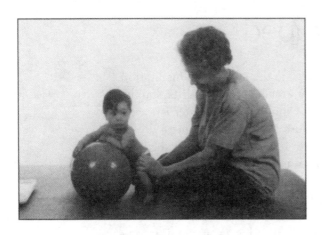

Figure 6.3.6. Option: The therapist performs the Prone to Sidelying With Lower-Extremity Weight-Bearing Progression facilitation on a peanut ball.

Option You can perform this same technique on a peanut ball (figure 6.3.6). The peanut ball is softer and higher than the bolster and thus is more comfortable and provides more trunk stability for some babies. The peanut may be easier for you to use because it is bigger and easier to move than the bolster.

Precautions

- Move slowly so the baby has time to adjust and adapt to the movements and the new positions.
- Maintain the alignment on the forward leg. The baby may tend to adduct and rotate the leg internally if the hip adductors are tight. The baby may tend to abduct and rotate the leg externally if the hip abductors are tight, the hip adductors are lengthened, or the baby has poor stability at the hip.
- Stabilize the baby's hips and both lower extremities during transitions between positions.
- Maintain the baby's trunk stability when the baby is in half-kneeling.

Component Goals

- Lateral flexion of the head and trunk with elongation on the weight-bearing side
- Lower-extremity dissociation
- Transitions between hip and knee extension and hip and knee flexion
- Weight bearing and weight shifts on the foot
- Sensory preparation of the foot
- Lower-extremity dissociation with weight bearing
- Active hip extension with knee flexion on the back leg
- Trunk extension over weight-bearing lower extremities

Functional Goals

- Maintain elongated side-sitting for play
- Transition from prone to half-kneeling in preparation for rising to stand

6.4 Climbing: Quadruped

The goal of this facilitation is to incorporate the quadruped facilitation techniques into climbing activities. Use an inclined wide bolster stabilized by a cube chair as the climbing surface. Climbing on a bolster is preferable to crawling on the floor because it is easier to control the baby's lower-extremity use and dissociation when climbing on the bolster. The bolster also is a novel idea and often is very motivating to babies.

Baby's Position The baby begins by standing at the bolster (figure 6.4.1) or in quadruped on the bolster (figure 6.4.3).

To participate in this facilitation, the baby must have some ability to bear weight on the upper extremities. However, do not underestimate the baby's ability to bear weight on the upper extremities. Abilities seem to increase when motivation is high, and climbing usually is a fun activity.

Therapist's Position Kneel behind the baby in a position to move with the baby.

Therapist's Hands and Movement

Initiation and Forward Progression
Place your hands on the baby's femurs near the knees, wrapping your hands around the baby's femurs so that your fingers are perpendicular to the femurs and your thumbs are parallel to the femurs (figures 6.4.1 and 6.4.3). Your *guiding hand* is on the weight-bearing leg; your *assisting hand* is on the unweighted leg.

Use your thumbs to facilitate the baby's hip extension by slightly pushing up toward the hip joint. Use your fingers to control the rotation of the baby's leg. Use your palms to control the abduction and adduction of each leg as well as knee flexion and extension.

If the baby starts in standing, use your *guiding hand* to shift the baby's weight laterally to one leg, and use your *assisting hand* to help the baby flex the unweighted leg at the hip and knee and place it on the bolster (figure 6.4.2).

When you place the baby's first leg on the bolster, use your *assisting hand* to stabilize the baby's flexed position as your *guiding hand* flexes the baby's extended leg and places it on the bolster (figure 6.4.3). When both legs are on the bolster, stabilize the baby's femurs with your fingers and press up and in with your thumbs to extend the baby's hips and shift the baby's weight forward onto the hands (figure 6.4.3).

Note: The first couple of times the babies climb up the bolster, they maintain strong hip flexion and keep their weight back so that little weight shifts onto the hands. This is normal but should change after several attempts to climb.

When the baby is stable, press forward and up with the thumb on your *guiding hand* to extend the baby's weight-bearing hip, and shift the baby's weight forward while simultaneously using your *guiding hand* to shift the baby's weight laterally on that hip. (In figure 6.4.4, the baby is bearing weight on the right hip. In figure 6.4.5, the baby is bearing

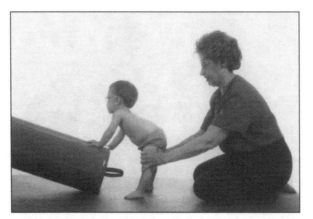

Figure 6.4.1. Climbing: Quadruped. Initiation and forward progression. With the baby standing at the bolster, the therapist places both hands on the baby's femurs near the knees, wrapping her hands around the baby's femurs so her fingers are perpendicular to the femurs and her thumbs are parallel to the femurs.

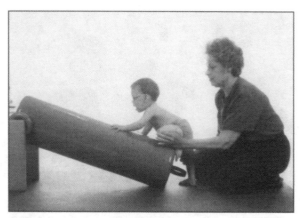

Figure 6.4.2. The therapist uses her *guiding hand* to shift the baby's weight laterally to the right leg and uses her *assisting hand* to help the baby flex the unweighted (left) leg at the hip and knee and place it on the bolster.

weight on the left hip. In each figure, the therapist presses forward with her thumb to extend the baby's weight-bearing hip.) This unweights the baby's other leg and enables the leg to move forward. When the baby's leg unweights, you may bring it into extension to increase the lower-extremity dissociation before you move it forward into flexion (figure 6.4.5, baby's right leg).

If the baby's leg does not move forward spontaneously, use your *assisting hand* to guide the baby's unweighted leg forward into hip and knee flexion and place the flexed leg in a weight-bearing position. (In figure 6.4.4, the therapist has unweighted the baby's left leg and flexed it forward, then placed it on the bolster in figure 6.4.5.)

Once the forward knee is in a weight-bearing position, use your thumb to extend the baby's hip subtly and shift the baby's weight laterally onto this leg.

Repeat the process several times as the baby shifts weight from side to side on alternate knees while climbing up the bolster. The weight shift is the critical element of this technique.

Rotation and Descent

When the baby reaches the top of the bolster, assist the baby to turn around by adducting the weight-bearing leg and guiding the baby into a side-sit position with your *guiding hand* (figure 6.4.6). Use your *assisting hand* to abduct and rotate the unweighted hip externally. Once the baby is in a stable side-sit position, move your *guiding hand* to the baby's trunk or pelvis and ensure the baby's stability (figure 6.4.7). Use your hands to rotate the baby's pelvis and trunk so the baby sits facing down the bolster (figure 6.4.8).

Note: Move one hand at a time when you are rotating the baby from quadruped to sitting. You must keep one hand on the baby at all times to ensure the baby's safety.

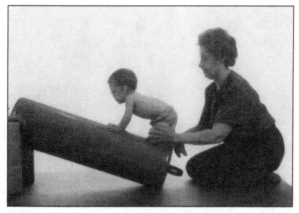

Figure 6.4.3. When placing the baby's first (left) leg on the bolster, the therapist uses her *assisting hand* to stabilize the baby's flexed position as her *guiding hand* flexes the baby's extended leg and places it on the bolster. When both legs are on the bolster, the therapist stabilizes the baby's femurs with her fingers and presses up and in with her thumbs to extend the baby's hips and shift the baby's weight forward onto the hands.

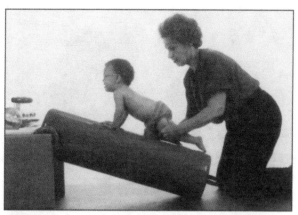

Figure 6.4.4. With the baby stable, the therapist presses forward and up with the thumb on her *guiding (right) hand* to extend the baby's hip and shift the baby's weight laterally. This unweights the baby's other leg. The therapist brings the unweighted (left) leg into extension to increase the lower-extremity dissociation before moving it forward into flexion.

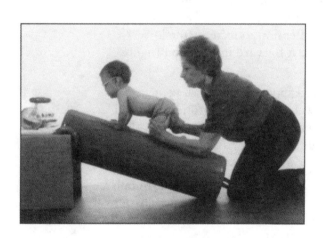

Figure 6.4.5. The therapist has placed the baby's flexed (left) knee on the bolster and is ready to use her thumb to extend the baby's left hip subtly and shift the baby's weight laterally again. The therapist extends the baby's right leg to increase the lower-extremity dissociation prior to moving it forward into flexion.

When the baby is facing down the bolster, move your hands, one at a time, to the baby's knees to extend the knees (figure 6.4.9). Once you have extended the baby's knees, slide the baby down the bolster (figure 6.4.10). When the baby reaches the end of the bolster, let the baby stand briefly (figure 6.4.11), then help the baby rotate and climb back up the bolster.

To slide down the bolster in this manner, the baby must have some trunk control to maintain the sitting posture independently. If the baby does not have sufficient trunk control to maintain this posture, do not attempt this step of the facilitation.

Component Goals

- Upper-extremity weight bearing and weight shifting
- Dynamic stability of the shoulder girdle muscles
- Forward progression over the upper extremities

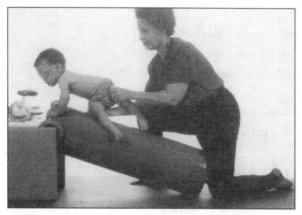

Figure 6.4.6. Rotation and descent. When the baby has reached the top of the bolster, the therapist assists the baby to turn around by adducting the weight bearing leg and guiding the baby into a side-sit position with her *guiding hand*, using her *assisting hand* to abduct and rotate the unweighted hip externally.

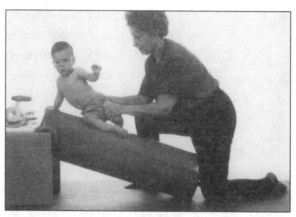

Figure 6.4.7. Once the baby is in a stable side-sit position, the therapist moves her *guiding hand* to the baby's pelvis and ensures the baby's stability.

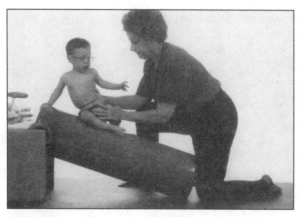

Figure 6.4.8. The therapist uses both hands to rotate the baby's pelvis and trunk so that the baby sits facing down the bolster.

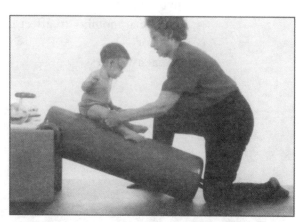

Figure 6.4.9. When the baby is facing down the bolster, the therapist moves her hands, one at a time, to the baby's knees to extend the knees.

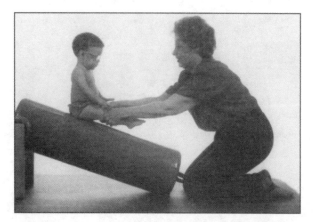

Figure 6.4.10. Having extended the baby's knees, the therapist slides the baby down the bolster.

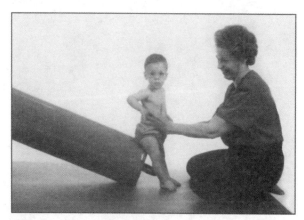

Figure 6.4.11. When the baby reaches the end of the bolster, the therapist lets the baby stand briefly before she helps the baby rotate and climb back up the bolster.

- Lower-extremity dissociation
- Reciprocal limb movements with trunk counterrotation
- Alternate elongation/activation of lower-extremity muscles
- Eccentric control of hip abductors and hip extensors during weight bearing
- Concentric control of hip adductors during weight bearing
- Concentric control of hip flexors, abductors, and external rotators during forward movement
- Elongation of hip flexors on the extended leg
- Elongation of the quadriceps on the flexed leg
- Lateral flexion of the trunk during the transition to sitting
- Pelvic rotation
- Trunk and pelvic control to maintain a sitting posture

Functional Goals
- Independence in climbing and crawling
- Cognitive enhancement with the ability to explore and affect the environment
- Functional mobility to affect the environment with goal-directed behavior
- Spatial awareness

6.5 Climbing: Bear Standing

The goal of this facilitation is to incorporate bear standing into climbing activities. Use an inclined wide bolster stabilized by a cube chair as the climbing surface.

The baby must have some ability to bear weight on the upper and lower extremities to participate in this facilitation.

Baby's Position The baby stands on the bolster with weight on both upper extremities and both lower extremities (figure 6.5.1). The baby is in a position to move forward.

Therapist's Position Kneel behind the baby in a position to move with the baby.

Therapist's Hands and Movement Place both of your hands on the baby's femurs near the knees, wrapping your hands around the baby's femurs so your fingers are perpendicular to the femurs and your thumbs are parallel to the femurs (figure 6.5.1).

Facilitate the baby's hip extension with your thumbs by slightly pushing up toward the hip joints. Your fingers control the rotation of the baby's hips while your palms control abduction and adduction of the hips as well as the flexion and extension of the knees.

Press forward and up with the thumb on your *guiding hand* to activate the baby's hip extensors, simultaneously using your *guiding hand* to shift the baby's weight laterally. In figure 6.5.1, the therapist's right thumb activates the baby's right hip extensor muscles. This unweights the baby's other (left) leg.

Use your *assisting hand* (left in figure 6.5.2) to guide the baby's unweighted leg forward, and place the foot in a weight-bearing position on the bolster (figure 6.5.2).

Once the forward foot is in a weight-bearing position, use your *assisting hand* to shift the baby's weight laterally to move the baby's weight onto this forward (left) leg. This unweights the baby's back (right) leg (figure 6.5.3).

Repeat the process several times as the baby shifts weight from side to side on alternate legs while progressing up the bolster. The weight shift is the critical element of this technique.

Note: It is important for the baby to have a goal or a reason to climb up the bolster (figure 6.5.4). As the baby reaches for the toy, be sure to stabilize the baby's legs with both of your hands.

Once at the top of the bolster, the baby may rotate the pelvis and trunk, sit down, and slide down the bolster as in figures 6.4.6 through 6.4.10.

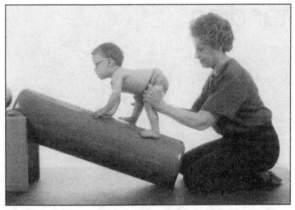

Figure 6.5.1. Climbing: Bear standing. The baby stands on the bolster with weight on both upper extremities and both lower extremities. The therapist places both hands on the baby's femurs near the knees, wrapping her hands around the baby's femurs so her fingers are perpendicular to the femurs and her thumbs are parallel to the femurs. The therapist presses forward and up with the thumb on her guiding (right) hand to activate the baby's hip extensors, simultaneously using the guiding hand to shift the baby's weight laterally. This will unweight the baby's other (left) leg.

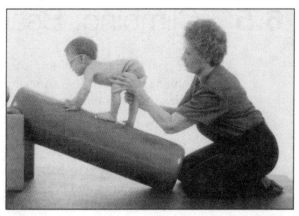

Figure 6.5.2. The therapist uses her *assisting (left) hand* to guide the baby's unweighted leg forward and place the foot in a weight-bearing position on the bolster.

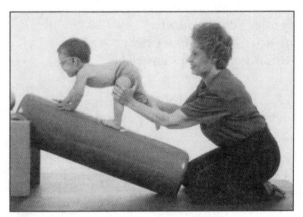

Figure 6.5.3. Once the forward foot is in a weight-bearing position, the therapist uses her *assisting (left) hand* to shift the baby's weight laterally to move the baby's weight onto this forward leg. This unweights the baby's back leg.

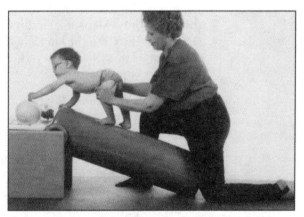

Figure 6.5.4. The therapist has placed a toy as a motivation for the baby to climb up the bolster. As the baby reaches for the toy, the therapist stabilizes the baby's legs with both hands.

Component Goals

- Upper-extremity weight bearing and weight shifting
- Dynamic stability of the shoulder girdle muscles
- Forward progression over the upper extremities
- Lower-extremity dissociation
- Reciprocal limb movements with trunk counterrotation
- Alternate elongation/activation of lower-extremity muscles

- Eccentric control of hip abductors and hip extensors during weight bearing
- Concentric control of hip adductors during weight bearing
- Concentric control of hip flexors, abductors, and external rotators during forward movement
- Elongation of the hamstrings
- Elongation of the gastrocnemius, soleus, and toe flexor muscles

Functional Goals

- Independence in climbing, crawling, and walking
- Cognitive enhancement with the ability to explore and affect the environment
- Perceptual awareness of heights

7. Floor Transitions

There are numerous sequences through which the baby can transition when playing on the floor. Some of the sequences enable the baby to play on the floor and others enable the baby to rise to standing from the floor. You can work on any or all of the sequences with the baby, depending on the baby's control. Although many of the sequences may appear to be too difficult for many babies, try them anyway. You will be helping the baby by facilitating the movement, and you will be stabilizing the baby with your hands throughout the movements.

7.1 Prone to Lower-Extremity Dissociation

The goal of this facilitation is for the baby to learn to transition from prone. Additional goals include mobility and control for lower-extremity dissociation; upper-extremity weight bearing; elongation of the hamstrings, toe flexors, quadriceps, and hip flexors; and activation of the hip and trunk extensors.

Baby's Position The baby lies prone or in forearm weight bearing on the floor with the hips extended.

Therapist's Position Kneel beside the baby.

Therapist's Hands and Movement Place your *guiding hand* under the baby's axilla onto the baby's trunk (figure 7.1.1). Place your *assisting hand* on the baby's far femur (figure 7.1.1).

Use your *guiding hand* to shift the baby's weight laterally into sidelying. At the same time, use your *assisting hand* to flex the baby's hip and knee and place the baby's foot on the floor (figure 7.1.2).

As the baby's weight shifts to one arm, the baby's other arm is free to reach. Use a toy that is interesting to the baby to facilitate the reach (figure 7.1.2). Check to make sure that the baby's bottom leg is extended at the hip and knee. The baby's leg must remain extended to keep the trunk muscles active.

Unilateral Weight Bearing
Continue to hold the baby's foot on the floor with your *assisting hand* while you move your *guiding hand* to the baby's knee (figure 7.1.3). Stabilize the baby's flexed leg with your *guiding hand*, and stabilize the baby's trunk with the forearm of your *guiding hand* (figure 7.1.3). Move your *assisting hand* to the baby's extended leg and place it over the baby's knee with your thumb on and parallel to the baby's femur (figure 7.1.3).

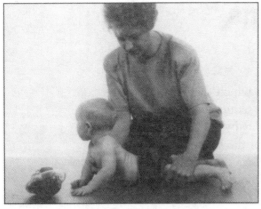

Figure 7.1.1. Prone to lower-extremity dissociation. The therapist places her *guiding hand* under the baby's axilla onto the baby's trunk, with her *assisting hand* on the baby's far femur.

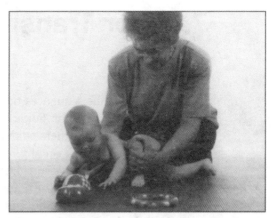

Figure 7.1.2. The therapist uses her *guiding hand* to shift the baby's weight laterally into sidelying, at the same time using her *assisting hand* to flex the baby's hip and knee and place the baby's foot on the floor. The baby's bottom leg remains extended at the hip and knee as the baby reaches for a toy with the now unweighted arm.

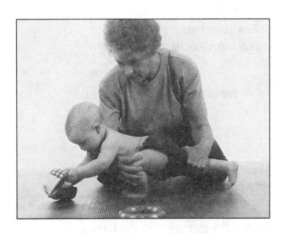

Figure 7.1.3. Unilateral weight bearing. The therapist moves her guiding hand under the baby's chest to the baby's flexed knee, stabilizing the baby's flexed leg with her guiding hand and stabilizing the baby's trunk with the forearm of her guiding hand. The therapist moves her assisting hand to the baby's extended leg and places it over the baby's knee, with her thumb on and parallel to the baby's femur. The therapist then shifts the baby's weight to the flexed leg by lifting the baby's extended leg and externally rotating it to neutral.

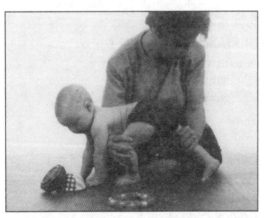

Figure 7.1.4. Bear-standing position. Keeping her hands in the same position as figure 7.1.3, the therapist uses both hands to shift the baby's weight diagonally, slightly forward and up, so that the baby's front knee begins to extend.

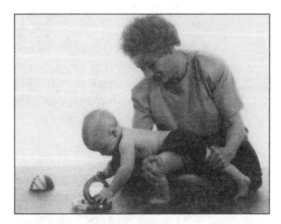

Figure 7.1.5. The therapist places the toes of the baby's back foot on the floor so the toes extend. The therapist shifts the baby's weight forward and backward in this position.

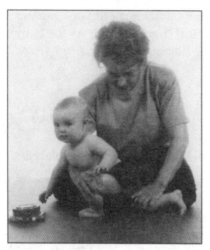 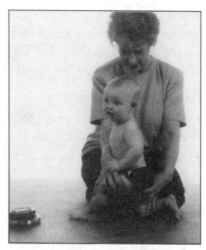

Figure 7.1.6. Half-kneeling. The therapist keeps her hands on the baby's legs and her forearm under the baby's trunk, using her *assisting hand* to flex the baby's back knee and place it on the floor.

Figure 7.1.7. When the baby's knee is on the floor, the therapist uses the forearm of her *guiding hand* to lift the baby's trunk to the vertical. As the baby's weight shifts to the back leg, the therapist spreads the fingers of her *assisting hand* to stabilize the baby's entire pelvis.

When both of your hands are in place, shift the baby's weight to the flexed leg by lifting the baby's extended leg and externally rotating it to neutral (figure 7.1.3). Support the baby's trunk with your forearm. Keep the baby's hip and knee extended and in line with the trunk. Use the thumb on your *assisting hand* to increase the baby's hip extension.

Bear-Standing Position
Keep your hands on the baby's legs and your forearm under the baby's trunk. Use both of your hands to shift the baby's weight diagonally, slightly forward and up, so that the front knee begins to extend (figure 7.1.4). Place the toes of the baby's back foot on the floor so the toes extend (figure 7.1.5).

You can shift the baby's weight forward and backward in this position. As the baby's weight shifts backward, the baby's toe flexors, gastrocnemius/soleus, and hamstrings of the back leg elongate. As the baby's weight shifts forward, the baby's gastrocnemius and quadriceps of the front leg elongate if you keep the baby's leg flexed (figure 7.1.5). The hamstrings elongate if you extend the baby's front knee.

Half-Kneeling
When the baby is in the bear-standing position (figure 7.1.5), keep your hands on the baby's legs and your forearm under the baby's trunk. Use your *assisting hand* to flex the baby's back knee and place it on the floor (figure 7.1.6). Keep the baby's toes on the floor when you flex the knee. Support the baby's trunk with your forearm and the baby's front leg with your *guiding hand* (figure 7.1.6).

When the baby's knee is on the floor, use the forearm of your *guiding hand* to lift the baby's trunk to the vertical (figure 7.1.7). As the baby's weight shifts to the back leg, spread the fingers of your *assisting hand* to stabilize the baby's entire pelvis (figure 7.1.7).

Precautions

- Keep your forearm under the baby's trunk to stabilize the baby's movements.
- Keep both of your hands on the baby's legs once you have placed them there.

Component Goals

- Elongation of the weight-bearing side
- Lower-extremity dissociation
- Flat-foot weight bearing on one foot
- Elongation of the toe flexors, gastrocnemius/soleus muscles, and hamstrings
- Preparation for push-off in gait
- Activation of all trunk muscles
- Activation of hip extensors and quadriceps
- Extension of the trunk on a stable pelvis

Functional Goals

- Transition from prone to bear standing
- Transition from bear standing to half-kneeling

7.2 Sitting to Quadruped to Kneeling

The goal of this facilitation is for the baby to learn to transition from sitting to quadruped and then to kneeling. Additional goals include trunk rotation, upper-extremity sideward protective extension, upper-extremity weight bearing and weight shifting, and hip extension with trunk extension.

Baby's Position The baby long-sits on the floor.

Therapist's Position Sit behind or beside the baby.

Therapist's Hands and Movement

Sitting to Quadruped

Place both of your hands on the lateral sides of the baby's trunk (figure 7.2.1), and rotate the baby's trunk so the baby's hand comes out into a sideward protective extension response (figure 7.2.2). Once the baby's hand is in a weight-bearing position, continue to rotate the baby's trunk around onto the arm until the baby assumes a quadruped position (figure 7.2.3). If the baby's weight-bearing arm becomes internally rotated as a result of the transition (figure 7.2.3), continue the movement until the opposite arm is in a weight-bearing position, then unweight the first arm so the baby can reposition it with external rotation. Let the baby reposition the arm independently. Do not reposition the arm for the baby; wait for the response.

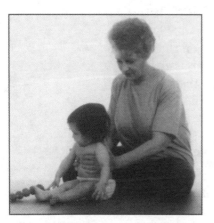

Figure 7.2.1. Sitting to quadruped. The therapist places both hands on the lateral sides of the baby's trunk.

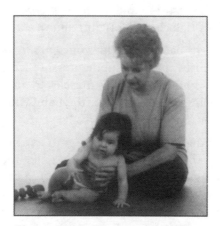

Figure 7.2.2. The therapist rotates the baby's trunk so the baby's hand comes out into a sideward protective extension response.

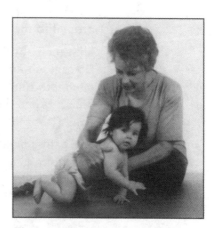

Figure 7.2.3. As a result of the transition, the baby's weight-bearing arm has become internally rotated. The therapist will continue the movement until the opposite arm is in a weight-bearing position, then unweight the first arm so that the baby can reposition it with external rotation.

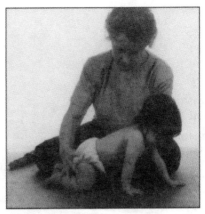

Figure 7.2.4. Quadruped to kneeling. With the baby in quadruped, the therapist keeps her *guiding hand* on the baby's rib cage and moves her *assisting hand* to the baby's posterior hip joints, spreading her thumb and fingers so they cover both hips. (In this photo, the therapist's *assisting-hand thumb* is on the baby's left hip and the *assisting-hand fingers* reach around to the baby's right hip and right femur.)

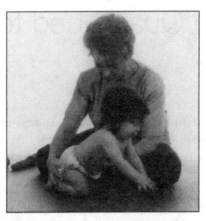

Figure 7.2.5. The therapist shifts the baby's weight backward with her *guiding hand* on the baby's rib cage, simultaneously applying subtle pressure with her *assisting hand* into the baby's gluteus maximus muscles to activate them. With the trunk stable, the baby begins to lift the hands from the floor.

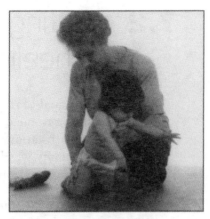

Figure 7.2.6. The therapist extends the baby's hips with her *assisting hand* while applying downward pressure into the knees and simultaneously guides the baby's trunk into extension with her *guiding hand.*

Quadruped to Kneeling

Once the baby is in quadruped, keep your *guiding hand* on the baby's rib cage and move your *assisting hand* to the baby's leg and posterior hip joints (figure 7.2.4). Spread your thumb and fingers so they cover both hips. (In figures 7.2.4 through 7.2.6, the therapist's *assisting-hand thumb* is on the baby's left hip and the *assisting-hand fingers* reach around to the baby's right hip and right femur.)

Shift the baby's weight backward with your *guiding hand* on the baby's rib cage, simultaneously applying subtle pressure with your *assisting hand* into the baby's gluteus maximus muscles to activate them (figure 7.2.5). When the baby's trunk is stable, the baby will begin to lift the hands from the floor (figure 7.2.5).

The baby's hand lifting is the signal for you to extend the baby's hips with your *assisting hand* and simultaneously guide the baby's trunk into extension with your *guiding hand* (figure 7.2.6). As you extend the baby's hips with your *assisting hand,* simultaneously apply downward pressure into the new base of support, the knees. Be careful not to overextend the baby's hips or trunk.

Precautions

- Keep both of your hands on the baby to stabilize the baby throughout the transition.
- Wait for the baby to make adjustments; do not do the adjustments for the baby.

- Do not overextend the baby's hips or trunk. Keep the hips directly below the shoulders.
- Do not force the baby up into kneeling; guide the movement.

Component Goals
- Trunk rotation
- Upper-extremity sideward protective extension
- Upper-extremity weight bearing and weight shifting
- Hip and knee flexion followed by hip extension with knee flexion
- Elongation of the quadriceps
- Activation of the gluteus maximus muscles
- Trunk extension on extended hips

Functional Goals
- Transition from sitting to quadruped
- Transition from quadruped to kneeling

7.3 Long-Sit to Quadruped With Forward Vaulting

The goals of this facilitation are to transition from sitting to quadruped, to elongate and activate the lower-extremity muscles, and to increase shoulder flexion and upper-extremity weight bearing. This transition is beneficial for babies who have tightness in their legs. Do not use this technique for babies with low muscle tone and hypermobility who keep their lower extremities in flexion, abduction, and external rotation.

Baby's Position The baby sits in a long-sitting or semilong-sitting position (figures 7.3.1 and 7.3.4).

Therapist's Position Sit or kneel behind the baby in a position that permits you to shift your weight forward with the baby.

Therapist's Hands and Movement Reach forward from behind the baby with your *assisting hand* and place one of the baby's legs in a ring position (figure 7.3.2, baby's right leg; figure 7.3.4, baby's left leg). Use your *assisting hand* to maintain the baby's leg in this position, and place your *guiding hand* on the baby's trunk (figure 7.3.2).

Use your *guiding hand* to extend and align the baby's trunk, then guide the baby's trunk forward from the hips as the baby reaches forward with both hands for a toy. The baby's reaching forward with both arms initiates the forward movement to quadruped. The baby's trunk and pelvis lean forward over the tibia of the flexed leg (figures 7.3.2 and 7.3.5).

As the baby reaches forward, move your *guiding hand* from the baby's trunk to the baby's forward leg. Position the leg so that the foot is in a weight-bearing position and the knee and hip flex (figure 7.3.3).

Use your *assisting hand* to stabilize the baby's back leg in external rotation (figures 7.3.3 and 7.3.5). Use the thumb of your *assisting hand* to lift the baby's hip, and shift the baby's weight forward (figures 7.3.6 and 7.3.7). As the baby reaches forward, the baby's trunk and pelvis move forward over the tibia of the back leg (figures 7.3.3, 7.3.5, and 7.3.6). Continue to shift the weight forward until the baby's arms assume a weight-bearing position (figures 7.3.6 and 7.3.7).

When weight transfers forward to the baby's arms, the baby's hip adductor and internal rotator muscles in both lower extremities elongate markedly (figure 7.3.3).

While keeping your *guiding hand* on the baby's forward leg, align the baby's back leg with your *assisting hand* by internally rotating the leg to neutral (figure 7.3.7). Adduct both legs and bring them into line with the trunk so they are not abducted.

You can use this three-point position as a transition to crawling or rising to stand. You also can reverse this three-point position to move back to sitting.

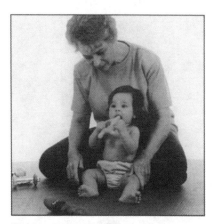

Figure 7.3.1. Long-sit to quadruped with forward vaulting. The baby sits in a long-sitting position.

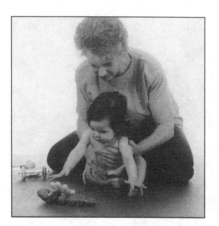

Figure 7.3.2. The therapist reaches forward from behind the baby with her *assisting (right) hand* and places the baby's right leg in a ring position. The therapist then uses her *assisting hand* to maintain the baby's leg in this position and places her *guiding hand* on the baby's trunk to extend and align the trunk and guide the baby's trunk forward from the hips. The baby reaches forward and initiates the forward movement to quadruped.

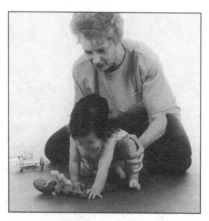

Figure 7.3.3. As the baby reaches forward, the therapist moves her *guiding hand* from the baby's trunk to the baby's forward leg and positions the leg so that the foot is in a weight-bearing position and the knee and hip flex. The therapist's *assisting hand* stabilizes the baby's back leg in external rotation.

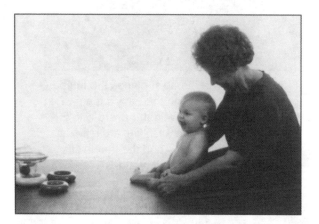

Figure 7.3.4. Semilong-sit to quadruped with forward vaulting. The baby sits in a semilong-sitting position with one knee extended and one knee flexed.

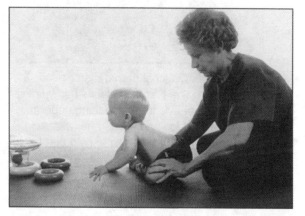

Figure 7.3.5. The therapist uses her *assisting (left) hand* to stabilize the baby's back leg in external rotation. As the baby reaches forward, the baby's trunk and pelvis move forward over the tibia of the back leg.

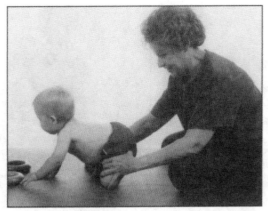

Figure 7.3.6. The therapist uses the thumb of her *assisting hand* to lift the baby's hip and shift the baby's weight forward over the tibia of the back leg.

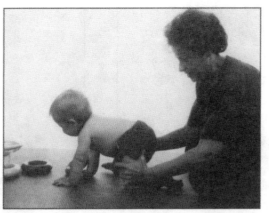

Figure 7.3.7. Keeping her *guiding hand* on the baby's forward leg, the therapist aligns the baby's back leg with her *assisting hand* by internally rotating the leg to neutral.

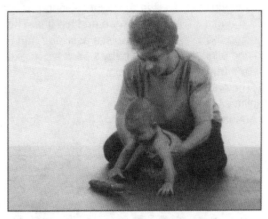

Figure 7.3.8. Optional preparation or modification. The therapist places her *guiding hand* on the baby's trunk, reaching under the baby's forward leg and placing her *assisting hand* on the baby's back leg to hold that leg in flexion and external rotation.

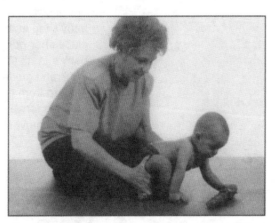

Figure 7.3.9. The therapist places the thumb of her *assisting hand* on the baby's femur, then shifts the baby's weight forward with the *guiding hand* while the *assisting hand* flexes the weight-bearing knee and the thumb lifts the baby's hip and pelvis forward.

Optional Preparation or Modification If the baby has difficulty controlling the legs during this transition, modify your hand placement so you can control both legs.

Place your *guiding hand* on the baby's trunk (figure 7.3.8). Reach under the baby's forward leg and place your *assisting hand* on the baby's back leg to hold that leg in flexion and external rotation (figures 7.3.8 and 7.3.9). Place the thumb of your *assisting hand* on the baby's femur (figure 7.3.9).

Shift the baby's weight forward with your *guiding hand* while your *assisting hand* flexes the weight-bearing knee and your thumb lifts the baby's hip and pelvis forward (figure 7.3.9).

Precaution Use this technique with babies who have tight hip adductors, not with babies who have excessive hip abduction, such as children with hypotonia or Down Syndrome.

Component Goals

- Elongation of the hip internal rotator muscles
- Elongation of the hip adductor muscles
- Elongation of the quadriceps on the flexed leg
- Lower-extremity dissociation
- Forward movement of the pelvis and trunk over the femurs
- Shoulder flexion with trunk extension and forward reaching
- Upper-extremity weight bearing and forward weight shifting

Functional Goals

- Transition from sitting to three point
- Transition from sitting to quadruped

7.4 Long-Sit to 5-Month Position

The goals of this facilitation are to increase the baby's trunk and lower-extremity mobility and to increase lower-extremity dissociation. The technique also prepares the foot and leg for weight bearing and weight shifting for rising to stand.

Baby's Position The baby long-sits on the floor with a neutrally aligned spine (or as close to neutral as possible) with hips flexed and knees extended (figure 7.4.1). If the baby cannot long-sit, you can modify this technique to semilong-sitting with slight knee flexion.

Therapist's Position Sit behind the baby in a position that permits you to shift your weight with the baby.

Therapist's Hands and Movement You will be performing this technique in several steps.

Preparation
Support and control the baby's trunk with your arms. With the *guiding hand*, reach forward from behind the baby's trunk to the baby's opposite leg (that is, your left hand to the baby's right knee) (figure 7.4.2). Reach under the baby's flexed leg, place your *assisting hand* on the baby's other leg, and extend the baby's knee (that is, your right hand to the baby's left knee) (figure 7.4.2).

With your *guiding hand,* pick up the baby's leg, flex the hip and knee, adduct it across the baby's other leg (figure 7.4.2), and place the baby's foot on the floor (figure 7.4.3). Maintain the knee extension of the baby's bottom leg with your *assisting hand.*

Once you have placed the baby's foot on the floor, push down through the baby's knee to the foot with your *guiding hand* to maintain the baby's foot in a weight-bearing position (figure 7.4.3).

Apply slight traction to the baby's bottom leg to extend the hip while maintaining the knee in extension (figure 7.4.4). The baby assumes a modified side-sitting position with elongation, rather than flexion, of the weight-bearing hip (figure 7.4.4).

Weight Shift Onto Flexed Leg
With the baby in the modified side-sitting position, use your *guiding hand* on the baby's flexed knee to adduct the leg slightly while applying forward traction to the femur, pelvis, and the trunk to shift additional weight onto the baby's foot. Your *guiding-hand arm* under the baby's arm provides support, helps lift the baby's trunk, and elongates the side as the baby's weight shifts forward (figure 7.4.5).

Your *assisting hand* lifts and applies backward traction to the baby's extended leg while externally rotating the baby's hip to neutral. This increases the weight shift of the trunk onto the flexed leg (figure 7.4.5).

If the baby's arm retracts when the weight shifts (figure 7.4.5), use the thumb of your *guiding hand* to flex the arm forward (figure 7.4.6).

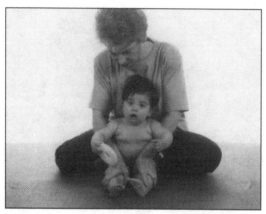

Figure 7.4.1. Long-sit to 5-month position: Preparation. The baby long-sits on the floor with a neutrally aligned spine, or as close to neutral as possible, with hips flexed and knees extended. The therapist supports and controls the baby's trunk with her arms.

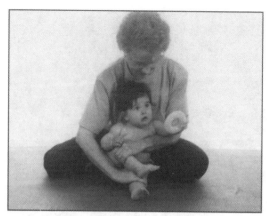

Figure 7.4.2. The therapist supports and controls the baby's trunk with her arms, while reaching forward from behind the baby's trunk with her *guiding (left) hand* to pick up the baby's right leg, flexing the hip and knee and adducting it across the baby's left leg. The therapist reaches under the baby's flexed leg to place the *assisting hand* on the baby's other leg to extend it.

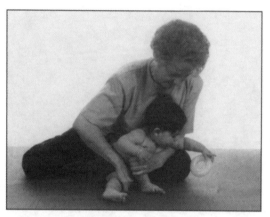

Figure 7.4.3. The therapist places the baby's right foot on the floor with the *guiding hand*, pushing down through the baby's knee to the foot to maintain the baby's foot in a weight-bearing position. The therapist uses her *assisting hand* to maintain the knee extension of the baby's bottom leg.

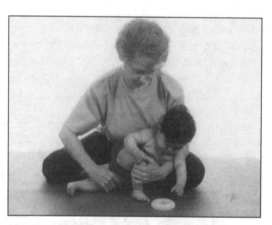

Figure 7.4.4. The therapist applies slight traction to the baby's bottom leg to extend the hip while maintaining the knee in extension. The baby assumes a modified side-sitting position with elongation, rather than flexion, of the weight-bearing hip.

Make sure you keep the fingers of your *guiding hand* on the baby's weight-bearing leg.

Take care to avoid excessive ankle dorsiflexion, which could cause the baby to collapse. Subtle backward traction of the baby's extended leg prevents excessive ankle dorsiflexion on the baby's forward flexed leg.

The resulting position should be one in which the baby bears weight on the foot of the flexed leg and both upper extremities. If the baby cannot bear weight on the upper extremities, your *guiding-hand arm* will support the baby's trunk (figure 7.4.6). Keep the baby's back leg lifted,

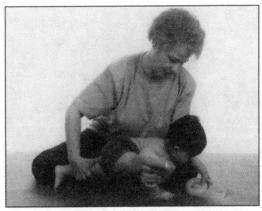

Figure 7.4.5. Weight shift onto flexed leg. The therapist uses her *guiding hand* on the baby's flexed knee to adduct the leg slightly while applying forward traction to the femur, pelvis, and the trunk to shift additional weight onto the baby's foot. The therapist's *guiding-hand arm* under the baby's arm provides support, helps lift the baby's trunk, and elongates the side as the baby's weight shifts forward. The therapist's *assisting hand* lifts and applies backward traction to the baby's extended leg while externally rotating the baby's hip to neutral, increasing the weight shift of the trunk onto the flexed leg.

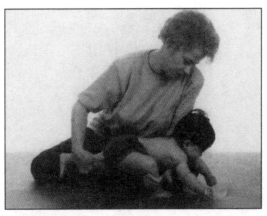

Figure 7.4.6. The therapist uses the thumb of her *guiding hand* to flex the baby's arm forward, which retracted when the weight shifted. The therapist keeps the fingers of her *guiding hand* on the baby's weight-bearing leg, supporting the baby's trunk with her *guiding-hand arm.*

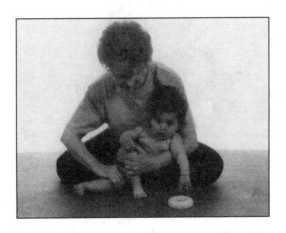

Figure 7.4.7. Return to modified side-sitting. The therapist uses her *assisting hand* to maintain the backward traction while internally rotating and lowering the baby's extended leg, her *guiding hand* and arm remaining in place during the transition to ensure the baby's safety and elongation of the weight-bearing side.

extended, and in line with the pelvis and trunk. The higher you lift the back leg while keeping it in line with the trunk, the more the knee of the forward leg extends.

Stabilize the baby with both hands, and facilitate subtle weight shifts forward and backward.

Return to Modified Side-Sitting
To return the baby to the modified side-sitting position, use your *assisting hand* to maintain the backward traction while you internally rotate and lower the baby's extended leg (figure 7.4.7).

Your *guiding hand and arm* must remain in place during the transition to ensure the baby's safety and elongation of the weight-bearing side.

Perform this entire sequence on both sides.

Precautions

- Your arm must support the baby's trunk when weight shifts onto the flexed leg.
- Make sure that the baby's trunk and pelvis both shift over the flexed leg.
- Do not abduct the baby's forward leg beside the trunk. This will cause the baby's pelvis to tilt anteriorly.
- Avoid excessive dorsiflexion, which can cause the baby to collapse. Keep the baby's back leg extended and tractioned backward to control dorsiflexion on the flexed leg.

Component Goals

- Marked lower-extremity dissociation
- Elongation of the trunk and hip muscles on the initial weight-bearing side
- Weight bearing on one foot
- Elongation of the heel cord and activation of the dorsiflexors
- Graded control of the quadriceps
- Hip and knee extension in line with the trunk
- Upper-extremity weight bearing and weight shifting

Functional Goals

- Transition from sitting to standing
- Ankle and foot preparation for gait

7.5 Prone to Standing

The goal of this facilitation is for the baby to learn to transition from prone to standing. Additional goals include mobility and control for lower-extremity dissociation, upper-extremity weight bearing, elongation and activation of the hip extensor muscles, weight shifts on the legs, and single-limb stance.

Baby's Position The baby lies prone or in forearm weight bearing on the floor with the hips extended.

Therapist's Position Kneel beside the baby.

Therapist's Hands and Movement

Prone to Quadruped
Place your *guiding hand* under the baby's axilla onto the baby's trunk (figure 7.5.1). Place your *assisting hand* on the baby's hips to extend the hips (figure 7.5.1).

Use your *guiding hand* to shift the baby's weight laterally into sidelying. At the same time, use your *assisting hand* to flex the baby's hip and knee and stabilize the pelvis (figure 7.5.2). Maintain that stability with your *assisting hand* by pushing the pelvis and hips down and backward.

Once the baby's legs are in the dissociated position, slide your *guiding hand* to the baby's flexed knee to keep it in line with the trunk and support the baby's trunk with your forearm (figure 7.5.3). Shift the baby's pelvis laterally onto the baby's flexed leg with your *assisting hand* while pushing the baby's weight backward (figure 7.5.3).

When the baby's weight shifts onto the flexed leg, reduce your backward pressure on the baby's pelvis and let the baby's extended leg flex so the baby comes to quadruped (figure 7.5.4).

Note: Keep your *guiding hand* on the baby's flexed knee and your forearm under the baby's trunk until the baby is in quadruped. Some babies have no or poor control of the hip muscles and often shoot into extension when attempting to come to quadruped.

Quadruped to Kneeling
Stabilize the baby's hips in quadruped with your *assisting hand* and move your *guiding hand* to the baby's rib cage (figure 7.5.4). Use your *guiding hand* to align the spine to neutral and shift the baby's weight backward as you continue to stabilize the baby's hips with your *assisting hand* (see figures 7.2.4 through 7.2.6).

Once the baby's weight has shifted backward, use your *guiding hand* to lift the baby's trunk slowly. Simultaneously extend the baby's hips by pressing into the baby's gluteus maximus with your *assisting hand* (figure 7.5.5). When the baby's gluteus maximus muscles activate, they help the baby elevate the trunk.

When the baby's hip extensors are active, the baby's ankles plantar flex (figure 7.5.5). If the baby's ankles are dorsiflexed, the baby is fixing with the hip flexors muscles. If ankle dorsiflexion occurs during the

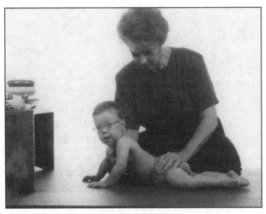

Figure 7.5.1. Prone to quadruped. The therapist places her *guiding hand* under the baby's axilla onto the baby's trunk and places her *assisting hand* on the baby's hips to extend the hips.

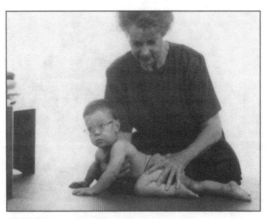

Figure 7.5.2. The therapist uses her *guiding hand* to shift the baby's weight laterally into sidelying. At the same time, the therapist uses her *assisting hand* to flex the baby's hip and knee and stabilize the pelvis, maintaining that stability with the *assisting hand* by pushing the pelvis and hips down and backward.

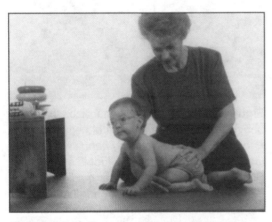

Figure 7.5.3. Once the baby's legs are in the dissociated position, the therapist slides her *guiding hand* to the baby's flexed knee to keep it in line with the trunk and supports the baby's trunk with her forearm. The therapist shifts the baby's pelvis laterally onto the baby's flexed leg with her *assisting hand* while pushing the baby's weight backward.

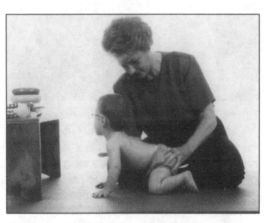

Figure 7.5.4. When the baby's weight shifts onto the flexed leg, the therapist reduces the backward pressure on the baby's pelvis and lets the baby's extended leg flex so the baby comes to quadruped. The therapist stabilizes the baby's hips in quadruped with her *assisting hand* while moving the *guiding hand* to the baby's rib cage and using it to align the spine to neutral and shift the baby's weight backward.

facilitation, increase the control provided by both of your hands to increase the baby's stability. It may take **several sessions** to reduce the baby's fixing with the hip flexors.

Kneeling to Half-Kneeling

With the baby's hips extended in kneeling, keep your hands in place and use both of them to shift the baby's weight laterally to the baby's leg that is close to you (figures 7.5.5 and 7.5.6). Your guiding hand helps the baby maintain trunk elevation during the weight shift, and

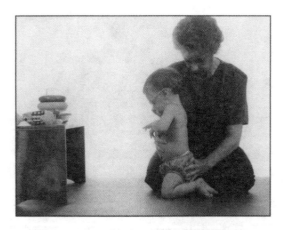

Figure 7.5.5. Quadruped to kneeling. Once the baby's weight has shifted backward, the therapist uses her *guiding hand* to lift the baby's trunk slowly, simultaneously extending the baby's hips by pressing into the baby's gluteus maximus with her *assisting hand*. Note the plantar flexion of the baby's ankles.

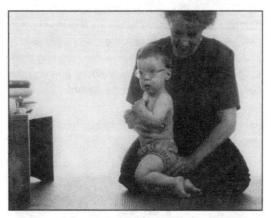

Figure 7.5.6. Kneeling to half-kneeling. With the baby's hips extended in kneeling, the therapist keeps her hands in place and uses both of them to shift the baby's weight laterally to the baby's leg that is close to her. Her *guiding hand* helps the baby maintain trunk elevation during the weight shift, and her *assisting hand* stabilizes the baby's pelvis and weight-bearing leg during the weight shift.

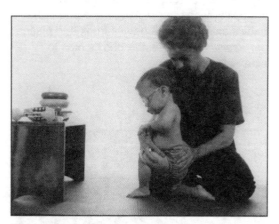

Figure 7.5.7. The therapist stabilizes the baby's trunk with the forearm of her *guiding hand* and slides her *guiding hand* to the baby's leg to lift and flex it until the foot is on the floor. She spreads the fingers of her *guiding hand* to stabilize the baby's trunk with her thumb and the baby's flexed leg with her fingers. Her *assisting hand* stabilizes the baby's pelvis and weight-bearing hip throughout the movement.

your assisting hand stabilizes the baby's pelvis and weight-bearing leg during the weight shift (figures 7.5.5 and 7.5.6).

When the baby's weight has shifted and the baby's far leg unweights, it should move forward into a weight-bearing position. If the baby has difficulty bringing the flexed leg forward, stabilize the baby's trunk with the forearm of your *guiding hand* and slide your *guiding hand* to the baby's leg, then lift and flex it and place the foot on the floor (figure 7.5.7). Spread the fingers of your *guiding hand* to stabilize the baby's trunk with your thumb and the baby's flexed leg with your fingers. Your *assisting hand* stabilizes the baby's pelvis and weight-bearing hip throughout the movement (figure 7.5.7).

Half-Kneeling to Standing
When the baby is stable in half-kneeling, place your *guiding hand* on the baby's trunk so your fingers control the lower rib cage and the abdominals (figure 7.5.8). Your hand placement helps the baby activate

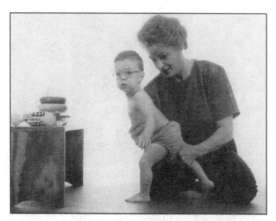

Figure 7.5.8. Half-kneeling to standing. The therapist places her *guiding hand* on the baby's trunk so her fingers control the lower rib cage and the abdominals. The therapist uses both hands to shift the baby's weight diagonally forward and up onto the forward leg, supporting the baby's trunk with her *guiding hand* and extending the baby's back hip and knee with her *assisting hand.*

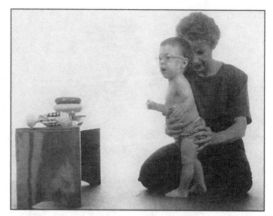

Figure 7.5.9. When the baby's weight is stable on the front leg, the therapist continues to support the baby's trunk with her *guiding hand*, then releases the back leg and moves her *assisting hand* to the baby's pelvis, stabilizing the baby in a symmetrical stance position. The therapist provides downward pressure with her hands on the baby's trunk and hips into the baby's feet to reinforce the somatosensory input for the new base of support at the feet.

the abdominals and helps prevent the baby from hyperextending the lumbar spine.

Use both of your hands to shift the baby's weight diagonally forward and up onto the forward leg (figure 7.5.8). As the baby's weight shifts forward, your *guiding hand* supports the baby's trunk, and your *assisting hand* extends the baby's back hip and knee (figure 7.5.8). Some babies may resist hip and knee extension of the back leg; extend the leg only as far as is comfortable for the baby.

When the baby's weight is stable on the front leg, continue to support the baby's trunk with your *guiding hand,* then release the back leg and move your *assisting hand* to the baby's pelvis (figure 7.5.9). Stabilize the baby in a symmetrical stance position. Provide downward pressure with your hands on the baby's trunk and hips into the baby's feet to reinforce the somatosensory input for the new base of support at the feet.

Options

Kneeling to Half-Kneeling
If the baby can use the upper extremities to assist with the transition from kneeling to half-kneeling, you can use the following technique.

When the baby is kneeling with the upper extremities on an elevated surface, place both of your hands across the baby's hips so that your thumbs press into the gluteus maximus and your fingers wrap around the femurs (figure 7.5.10). Use both of your hands to align the baby's pelvis and trunk over the femurs.

Stabilize the baby's hips with both of your hands and shift the baby's weight laterally over one leg. As one leg unweights, it will respond with

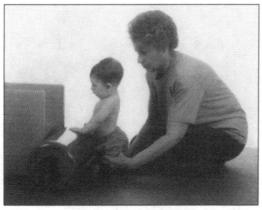

Figure 7.5.10. Kneeling to half-kneeling. With the baby kneeling with the upper extremities on an elevated surface, the therapist places both hands across the baby's hips so that her thumbs press into the gluteus maximus and her fingers wrap around the femurs, using both hands to align the baby's pelvis and trunk over the femurs.

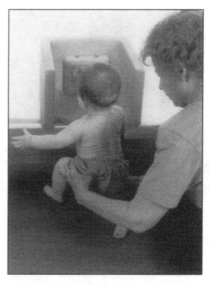

Figure 7.5.11. The therapist stabilizes the baby's hips with both hands and shifts the baby's weight laterally over the right leg. As the left leg unweights, it responds with forward flexion of the hip and knee, and the baby assumes a half-kneel position.

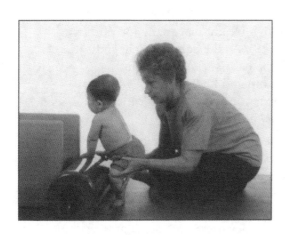

Figure 7.5.12. With the baby's left leg forward in a weight-bearing position, the therapist uses both hands to shift the baby's weight diagonally forward and up to standing, spreading her fingers to stabilize the baby's left femur, knee, and lower leg to give more control of the forward leg.

forward flexion of the hip and knee and assume a half-kneel position (figure 7.5.11).

Once the one leg is forward in a weight-bearing position, use both of your hands to shift the baby's weight diagonally forward and up to standing (figure 7.5.12). If the baby needs more control of the forward leg, you can spread your fingers to stabilize the baby's femur, knee, and lower leg (figure 7.5.12).

Half-Kneeling to Standing
If the baby needs help stabilizing the forward flexed leg, place your *guiding hand* on the front leg with your forearm on the baby's trunk (figure 7.5.13).

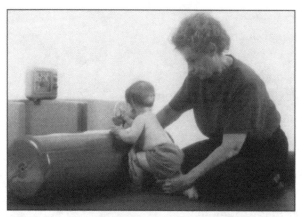

Figure 7.5.13. Half-kneeling to standing. To help the baby stabilize the forward flexed leg, the therapist places her *guiding hand* on the front leg and her forearm on the baby's trunk, then moves her *assisting hand* to the baby's leg that is close to her, grasping the baby's femur so that her thumb is parallel to the baby's femur.

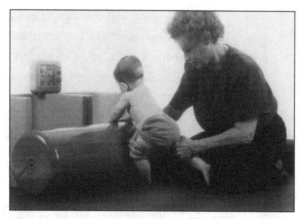

Figure 7.5.14. The therapist uses both hands to shift the baby's weight diagonally forward and up, supporting the baby's forward leg with her *guiding hand* and extending the baby's back hip and knee with her *assisting hand*.

Move your *assisting hand* to the baby's leg that is close to you. Grasp the baby's femur so your thumb is parallel to the baby's femur (figure 7.5.13).

Use both of your hands to shift the baby's weight diagonally forward and up (figure 7.5.14). As the baby's weight shifts forward, your *guiding hand* supports the baby's forward leg, and your *assisting hand* extends the baby's back hip and knee (figure 7.5.14). Some babies may resist hip and knee extension of the back leg; extend the leg only as far as is comfortable for the baby.

When the baby's weight is stable on the front leg, move the back leg into a weight-bearing position. Then move your *assisting hand* to the baby's pelvis. When the baby is again stable, move your *guiding hand* to the baby's pelvis and stabilize the baby in a symmetrical position.

Precautions

- Keep your hands on the baby to provide stability to the baby throughout all of the transitions.
- Wait for the baby to make adjustments after each weight shift; do not do the adjustments for the baby.

Component Goals

- Lateral weight shifts with elongation of the weight-bearing side in prone to sidelying and kneeling to half-kneeling
- Lateral righting of the unweighted side in prone to sidelying and kneeling to half-kneeling
- Upper-extremity weight bearing and weight shifting
- Lower-extremity dissociation with hip and knee flexion on one side, and with hip and knee extension on the other side
- Hip extension with knee flexion

- Elongation of the quadriceps and hip flexors
- Activation of the hip extensor and hip abductor muscles
- Trunk extension on extended hips
- Dissociation of the lower extremities under the trunk
- Transitions between ankle plantar flexion and dorsiflexion
- Elongation of the ankle dorsiflexor muscles

Functional Goals
- Transition from prone to quadruped
- Transition from quadruped to kneeling
- Transition from kneeling to half-kneeling to standing

8. Sitting on Lap

8.1 Upper-Extremity Forward Reaching While Sitting

The goal of this facilitation is for the baby to learn to reach forward with the arms when sitting. Additional goals include trunk control and balance for sitting and for reaching, and trunk extension with hip flexion and shoulder flexion.

Baby's Position The baby sits on your leg.

Therapist's Position Sit on the floor with one of your legs flexed and the other extended in front of you (figure 8.1.1).

Therapist's Hands and Movement Place both of your hands laterally on the baby's trunk, especially on the rib cage, to support and stabilize the baby (figure 8.1.1). Apply gentle pressure with your thumbs to help the baby extend the trunk. Move your index fingers to the baby's arms slightly above the elbows and bring the baby's arms into flexion and adduction against the baby's sides (figure 8.1.1).

Place a ball or a peanut ball in front of the baby to give the baby a target for which to reach. Make sure that the ball is of a height that enables the baby to keep the trunk erect when the arms reach forward

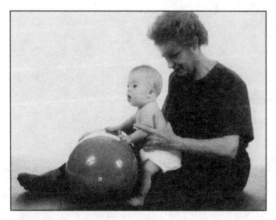

Figure 8.1.1. Upper-extremity forward reaching while sitting. The therapist sits on the floor with her left leg flexed and the other extended in front of her, using her right foot to stabilize the ball. The therapist places both hands laterally on the baby's trunk, applying gentle pressure with her thumbs to help the baby extend the trunk. The therapist moves her index fingers to the baby's arms slightly above the elbows to bring the baby's arms into flexion and adduction against the baby's sides.

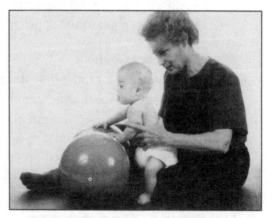

Figure 8.1.2. The therapist stabilizes the baby's hands on the ball with her fingers on the baby's arms, pressing the baby's arms (and thus the baby's hands) into the ball.

(figure 8.1.1). You can use your foot to stabilize the ball for the baby (figure 8.1.1, therapist's right foot).

When the baby's hands are on the ball, stabilize them there with your fingers on the baby's arms, then use your hands to press the baby's arms, thus the baby's hands, into the ball (figure 8.1.2). This simulates a weight-bearing experience for the baby. Try to keep the baby's elbows extended.

Suggestions

- Use singing to engage the baby.
- Encourage the baby's caregiver to sit in front of the baby to facilitate the baby's head/visual responses.
- Hold or place a suction-cup toy on the ball to engage the baby's attention and encourage the baby's reaching.

Precautions

- Your hands must be firm enough to stabilize the baby but light enough to enable the baby's trunk muscles to work.
- Maintain the baby's erect sitting posture with flexed hips throughout the movement.
- Stabilize the ball with your foot so the ball does not roll away when the baby pushes on the ball.

Component Goals

- Trunk extension with hip and knee flexion
- Shoulder flexion
- Elbow and wrist extension
- Upper-extremity weight bearing and pushing
- Proprioception in the upper extremities

Functional Goals

- Preparation for independent sitting
- Preparation for upper-extremity reaching
- Preparation for upper-extremity weight bearing, which is needed for transitional movements
- Preparation for forward protective extension

8.2 Lateral Weight Shifts/Lateral Righting: "Happy Face"

The goals of this facilitation are for the baby to develop the ability to shift weight laterally and use lateral righting reactions when sitting. Additional goals include appropriate registration of changing sensory feedback; appropriate postural responses and balance reactions to displacement of the center of mass; anticipation of balance requirements; eccentric elongation of hip, trunk, and neck muscles on the weight-bearing side; concentric activation of hip, trunk, and neck muscles on the unweighted side; and activation of upper-extremity sideward protective extension responses.

This technique is titled "Happy Face" because your hands move in an arc that resembles a happy face, that is, upward elongation of the baby's trunk at the end of each weight shift.

Baby's Position The baby sits across your lap.

Therapist's Position Long-sit on the floor (figure 8.2.1), or sit on a bench or ball with your hips flexed to 90°.

Therapist's Hands Place your hands on the front and back of the baby's trunk, and spread your fingers so you can hold the baby's rib cage (figures 8.2.1 and 8.2.4). Your hands should be firm but not hard.

Movement With your hands firmly but gently on the baby, align the baby's trunk to neutral on the sagittal plane (or as close to neutral as possible). Do not let the baby's trunk flex or hyperextend.

With an arc-like movement of your arms and hands and a forward weight shift of your body, shift the baby's weight laterally onto the far hip (figures 8.2.2 and 8.2.4). As you shift your weight forward, simultaneously use your fingers to elongate the baby's side (figure 8.2.2). Make sure you shift the weight in the baby's pelvis as well as in the rib cage. Never shift the rib cage over the pelvis without the pelvis moving. This will cause elongation of the muscles between the rib cage and the pelvis and will lead to trunk instability.

Once you shift the baby's weight to the side, **wait** for the baby to respond with a lateral righting reaction of the head, neck, and trunk (figures 8.2.3 through 8.2.5) and possibly abduction of the unweighted leg (figures 8.2.4 and 8.2.5).

Shift the baby's weight laterally to the other side with an arc-like movement of your arms and hands and a backward weight shift of your body (figures 8.2.3 and 8.2.5). Shift the baby's weight onto the hip by elongating the baby's side with your thumbs and/or the heels of your hands. Make sure you shift the weight in the baby's pelvis as well as in the rib cage. Never shift the rib cage over the pelvis without the pelvis moving.

Repeat the lateral weight shift several times in both directions.

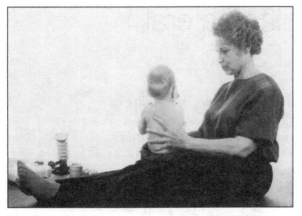

Figure 8.2.1. Lateral weight shifts/lateral righting: "Happy face." The therapist long-sits on the floor with hips flexed to 90°; the baby sits across her lap. The therapist places her hands on the front and back of the baby's trunk, spreading her fingers to hold the baby's rib cage and aligning the baby's trunk to neutral on the sagittal plane.

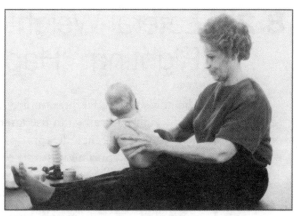

Figure 8.2.2. The therapist shifts the baby's weight laterally onto the far hip with an arc-like movement of her arms and hands and a forward weight shift of her body, simultaneously using her fingers to elongate the baby's left side.

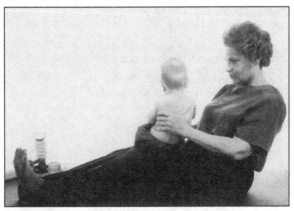

Figure 8.2.3. The therapist shifts the baby's weight laterally to the other side with an arc-like movement of her arms and hands and a backward weight shift of her body, elongating the baby's side with her thumbs and the heels of her hands.

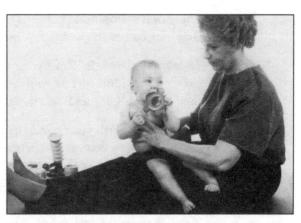

Figure 8.2.4. As the baby's weight shifts to the side, the baby responds with a lateral righting reaction of the head, neck, and trunk.

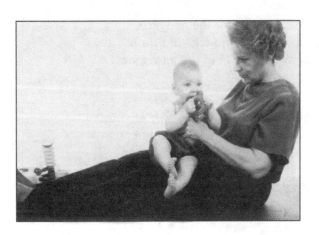

Figure 8.2.5. Sometimes the baby also responds to the weight shift with abduction of the unweighted leg.

Suggestions

- Sing to engage the baby during the weight shifts.
- Encourage the baby's caregiver to sit in front of the baby, and move from side to side with the baby to facilitate the baby's head/visual responses.
- Move a toy from side to side to facilitate head righting.

Precautions

- Your hands must be firm enough to make the baby feel comfortable, but not so hard as to cause discomfort to the baby.
- Always shift the pelvis with the rib cage.
- Move only laterally on the frontal plane. Do not rotate the baby.
- Wait for the baby to respond with lateral righting.

Component Goals

- Elongation of muscles on the weight-bearing side
- Eccentric activation of the hip, trunk, and neck muscles on the weight-bearing side
- Concentric activation of the hip, trunk, and neck muscles on the unweighted side
- Sensory stimulation through the tactile, proprioceptive, visual, and vestibular systems
- Stimulation of the righting reactions through the detection of the sensory feedback
- Muscle activation for lateral righting reactions of the head and trunk

Functional Goals

- Preparation for all lateral weight shifts
- Preparation for lateral weight shifts for transitional movements
- Ability to adapt and respond to incoming sensory stimulation

8.3 Lateral Weight Shifts/Lateral Righting: Elongation of Scapulo-Humeral Muscles

The goal of this facilitation is to elongate the muscles between the scapula and humerus (latissimus dorsi, teres major, and long head of the triceps) while activating the lateral righting reactions. Additional goals include all of those for lateral weight shifts listed in 8.2, Lateral Weight Shifts/Lateral Righting: "Happy Face."

Baby's Position   The baby sits across your lap.

Therapist's Position   Long-sit on the floor (figure 8.3.1), or sit on a bench or ball with your hips flexed to 90°.

Therapist's Hands   Place your *guiding hand* on the baby's anterior rib cage (figure 8.3.1). Spread your fingers so that you can hold the baby's rib cage (figures 8.3.1 and 8.3.3). Your hand should be firm, but do not squeeze.

Reach your *assisting hand* behind the baby's back, place it on the baby's far arm over the elbow, and externally rotate the humerus (figures 8.3.1 and 8.3.4). The arm of your *assisting hand* contacts the baby's back (figure 8.3.4).

Use your *guiding hand* and the arm of your *assisting hand* to align the baby's trunk to neutral on the sagittal plane (or as close to neutral as possible). When you have aligned the baby's trunk, shift the baby's weight laterally to one hip.

Movement

Weight Shift Away From You

Shift the baby's weight away from you by simultaneously shifting your weight forward, applying an arc-like movement to the baby's trunk with your *guiding hand*, and abducting and flexing the baby's far arm overhead with your *assisting hand* (figures 8.3.2 and 8.3.5). Maintain the arm of your *assisting hand* on the baby's back to assist the baby with trunk extension. Shoulder flexion with external rotation helps elongate the weight-bearing side by elongating the latissimus dorsi.

Use the fingers of your *guiding hand* to elongate the baby's side as you shift the baby's weight laterally onto one hip. Make sure you shift the weight in the baby's pelvis as well as in the rib cage. Never shift the rib cage over the pelvis without the pelvis moving. This will cause elongation of the muscles between the rib cage and the pelvis and will lead to trunk instability.

If there is muscle tightness between the scapula and humerus, shoulder flexion may cause the scapula to wing laterally away from the rib cage. If this happens, flex the baby's arm only to the point where the scapula **begins** to wing laterally. Place the fingers of your *guiding hand* on the lateral border of the baby's scapula and gently stabilize it on the rib

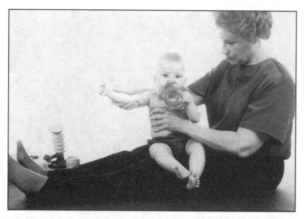

Figure 8.3.1. Lateral weight shifts/lateral righting: Elongation of scapulo-humeral muscles. The therapist long-sits on the floor with hips flexed to 90°; the baby sits across her lap. The therapist places her *guiding hand* on the baby's anterior rib cage, spreading her fingers to hold the baby's rib cage. The therapist reaches her *assisting hand* behind the baby's back, placing it on the baby's far arm over the elbow and externally rotating the humerus. The therapist's *guiding hand* and the arm of her *assisting hand* align the baby's trunk to neutral on the sagittal plane.

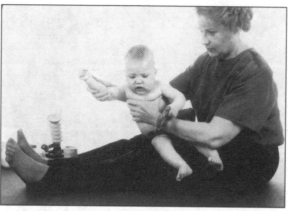

Figure 8.3.2. The therapist shifts the baby's weight away from her by shifting her weight forward. At the same time, the therapist applies an arc-like movement to the baby's trunk with her *guiding hand* and externally rotates, abducts, and flexes the baby's far arm overhead with her *assisting hand*, maintaining the arm of her *assisting hand* on the baby's back to assist the baby with trunk extension.

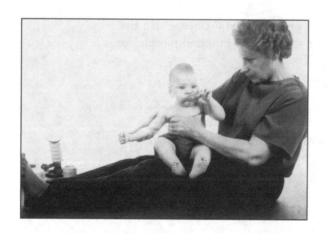

Figure 8.3.3. The therapist shifts the baby's weight toward her by simultaneously shifting her weight backward, applying an arc-like movement to the baby's trunk with her *guiding hand*, and lowering the baby's far arm with her *assisting hand* while maintaining the arm of her *assisting hand* on the baby's back to assist the baby with trunk extension. The therapist uses the thumb of her *guiding hand* to elongate the baby's side gently as she shifts the baby's weight laterally onto one hip.

cage as you flex the baby's arm slightly higher during the weight shift. Do not restrict the scapula totally. Permit it to move slightly with the humerus. The goal is to establish the normal 2:1 scapulo-humeral rhythm in which the scapula moves 1° for every 2° of humeral movement.

Weight Shift Toward You
Shift the baby's weight toward you by simultaneously shifting your weight backward, applying an arc-like movement to the baby's trunk with your *guiding hand*, and lowering the baby's far arm with your *assisting hand* (figure 8.3.3). Maintain the arm of your *assisting hand* on the baby's back to assist the baby with trunk extension.

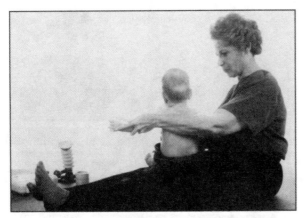

Figure 8.3.4. The therapist turns the baby in the other direction to elongate the scapulo-humeral muscles on the baby's left side. The therapist's *assisting-hand arm* contacts the baby's back to support the trunk preparatory to the weight shift.

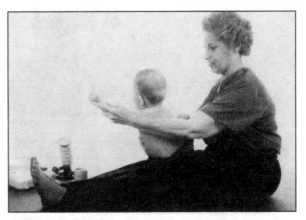

Figure 8.3.5. Back view of the therapist's *assisting hand* abducting and flexing the baby's far arm overhead during a weight shift away from the therapist.

Use the thumb of your *guiding hand* to elongate the baby's side gently as you shift the baby's weight laterally onto one hip. Make sure you shift the weight in the baby's pelvis as well as in the rib cage. Never shift the rib cage over the pelvis without the pelvis moving. This will cause elongation of the muscles between the rib cage and the pelvis and will lead to trunk instability.

Repeat the weight shift and elongation process several times. Turn the baby in the other direction to elongate the scapulo-humeral muscles of the other arm (figures 8.3.4 and 8.3.5).

Suggestion Sing to engage the baby during the weight shifts.

Precautions
- Shift your body forward and backward with the baby's weight shift. This helps facilitate the baby's weight shift.
- Hold the baby's rib cage firmly, but gently. Do not squeeze the rib cage.
- Flex, abduct, and externally rotate the shoulder simultaneously with the lateral weight shift.
- Always shift the pelvis with the rib cage.
- Move only laterally on the frontal plane. Do not rotate the baby.
- Wait for the baby to respond with lateral righting.
- If you stabilize the scapula, do not totally restrict it. Permit it to move slightly with the humerus.

Component Goals
- Elongation of muscles on the weight-bearing side
- Emphasis on elongation of the muscles between the scapula and humerus
- Eccentric activation of the hip, trunk, and neck muscles on the weight-bearing side

- Concentric activation of the hip, trunk, and neck muscles on the unweighted side
- Sensory stimulation through the tactile, proprioceptive, visual, and vestibular systems
- Stimulation of the righting reactions through the detection of the sensory feedback
- Muscle activation for lateral righting reactions of the head and trunk

Functional Goals
- Preparation for all lateral weight shifts
- Elongation of scapulo-humeral muscles to enable for normal 2:1 scapulo-humeral rhythm
- Upper-extremity preparation for reaching and sideward protective extension

8.4 Lateral Weight Shifts With Shoulder Girdle Depression

The goal of these facilitation techniques is to elongate the muscles that elevate the shoulders and hyperextend the neck (upper trapezius and levator scapulae) while activating the lateral righting reactions. Additional goals include all of those for lateral weight shifts listed in facilitation 8.2, Lateral Weight Shifts/Lateral Righting: "Happy Face."

Baby's Position The baby sits across your lap.

Therapist's Position Long-sit on the floor (figure 8.4.1), or sit on a bench or ball with your hips flexed to 90°.

Therapist's Hands Place your *guiding hand* on the baby's near humerus so the palm of your hand and your fingers hold the humerus. Your index finger rests on the baby's shoulder (figures 8.4.2 and 8.4.4).

Reach your *assisting hand* behind the baby's back, place it on the baby's far arm over the elbow, and externally rotate the humerus (figures 8.4.1 and 8.4.2). The arm of your *assisting hand* contacts the baby's trunk (figure 8.4.2).

Movement Use the arm of your *assisting hand* to extend the baby's trunk and align it to neutral on the sagittal plane (or as close to neutral as possible). Externally rotate the baby's humeri to facilitate additional trunk extension.

When you have aligned the baby's trunk, shift the baby's weight laterally to one hip.

Weight Shift Toward You
Shift the baby's weight toward you by shifting your weight backward while you simultaneously use your *guiding hand* and arm to apply traction to abduct and flex the baby's near arm (figure 8.4.3). As the baby's weight shifts to the near hip, lower the baby's far arm with your *assisting hand* to help facilitate lateral righting of the head and trunk on the unweighted side (figure 8.4.3). Maintain the forearm of your *assisting hand* on the baby's back to assist the baby with trunk extension.

Make sure you shift the weight in the baby's pelvis as well as in the rib cage. Never shift the rib cage over the pelvis without the pelvis moving. This will cause elongation of the muscles between the rib cage and the pelvis and will lead to trunk instability.

Weight Shift Away From You
Shift the baby's weight away from you by shifting your weight forward while you simultaneously use your *assisting hand* and arm to apply traction to rotate externally, abduct, and flex the baby's far arm (figure 8.4.5). This arm movement with the weight shift elongates the baby's side. Maintain the arm of your *assisting hand* on the baby's back to assist the baby with trunk extension.

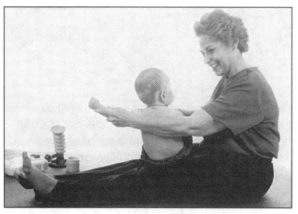

Figure 8.4.1. Lateral weight shifts with shoulder-girdle depression. The therapist long-sits on the floor with hips flexed to 90°; the baby sits across her lap. The therapist places her *guiding hand* on the baby's near humerus so the palm of her hand and fingers hold the humerus and the index finger rests on the baby's shoulder. The therapist reaches her *assisting hand* behind the baby's back, placing the *assisting hand* on the baby's far arm over the elbow to rotate the humerus externally. She uses her *assisting-hand arm* to extend the baby's trunk and align it to neutral in the sagittal plane.

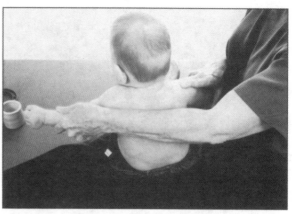

Figure 8.4.2. Closer view of the therapist's *guiding hand* on the baby's near humerus with the palm of her hand and her fingers holding the humerus, her index finger resting on the baby's shoulder. The therapist's *assisting hand* is on the baby's far elbow, externally rotating the humerus, and the *assisting-hand arm* is in contact with the baby's trunk.

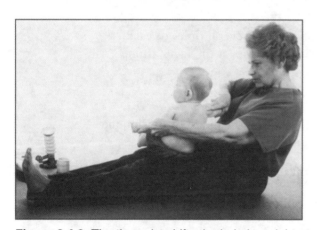

Figure 8.4.3. The therapist shifts the baby's weight toward herself by shifting her weight backward while simultaneously using her *guiding hand* and arm to apply traction to rotate externally, abduct, and flex the baby's near arm. As the baby's weight shifts to the near hip, the therapist lowers the baby's far arm with her *assisting hand*, keeping her *assisting-hand* forearm on the baby's back to assist the baby with trunk extension.

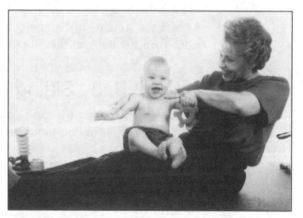

Figure 8.4.4. Front view of the weight shift toward the therapist, showing the position of the *guiding hand* as the therapist applies traction to abduct and flex the baby's near arm. The therapist lowers the baby's far arm with her *assisting hand* to help facilitate lateral righting of the head and trunk on the unweighted side.

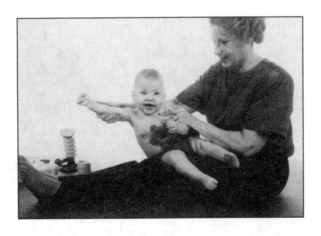

Figure 8.4.5. Front view of the weight shift away from the therapist. The therapist uses her *guiding hand* to apply subtle pressure diagonally downward from the baby's near (left) shoulder toward the far (right) hip. The therapist's *assisting hand* and arm apply traction to rotate externally, abduct, and flex the baby's far arm.

Simultaneously use your *guiding hand* to apply subtle pressure diagonally downward from the baby's near shoulder toward the far hip. (In figure 8.4.5, the therapist applies pressure from the baby's left shoulder to the baby's right hip.) This helps shift the baby's weight to the far hip and helps facilitate lateral flexion of the trunk on the unweighted side. The diagonal pressure also helps increase the somatosensory feedback from the new base of support.

Make sure you shift the weight in the baby's pelvis as well as in the rib cage. Never shift the rib cage over the pelvis without the pelvis moving. This will cause elongation of the muscles between the rib cage and the pelvis and will lead to trunk instability.

Repeat the weight shift and elongation process several times to each side. Turn the baby in the other direction and repeat the facilitation.

Option: Baby Sitting on the Floor

If the baby is too big to sit on your lap, you can facilitate this technique with the baby sitting on the floor (figure 8.4.6).

Baby's Position The baby long-sits on the floor.

Therapist's Position Sit behind the baby in a position to shift your weight with the baby.

Therapist's Hands Place your hands on the baby's arms over the elbows so the palms of your hands and your fingers hold the baby's arms. Your index fingers rest on the baby's shoulders (figure 8.4.6). Abduct and externally rotate both arms to facilitate trunk extension and align the trunk to neutral (or as close to neutral as possible). Apply slight downward pressure with your index fingers to depress the baby's shoulders and to direct somatosensory input into the base of support.

Movement While maintaining both arms in abduction and external rotation with slight shoulder depression, apply traction to one arm in a **lateral and upward** direction. Lower the other arm slightly (figure 8.4.6).

The traction is slow but strong enough to produce a weight shift in the trunk and pelvis. The pelvis must move over the femur. The weight-

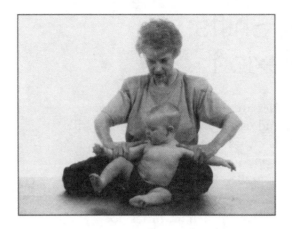

Figure 8.4.6. Option: Baby sitting on the floor. The therapist's hands are on the baby's arms over the elbows so the palms of her hands and her fingers hold the baby's arms, with her index fingers resting on the baby's shoulders. The therapist abducts and externally rotates both arms, applying slight downward pressure with her index fingers. While maintaining both arms in abduction and external rotation with slight shoulder depression, the therapist applies traction to the baby's left arm in a lateral and upward direction, lowering the right arm slightly. The baby's unweighted leg abducts to balance the weight shift.

bearing side is the elongated side. The unweighted side laterally flexes as a response to elongation on the weight-bearing side. The unweighted leg may abduct to balance the weight shift (figure 8.4.6).

Perform the weight shift to each side.

Suggestions

- Sing to engage the baby during the weight shifts.
- Sit with the baby facing a mirror.

Precautions

- Maintain the baby's trunk extension with your *assisting forearm* during the weight shifts.
- Make sure you externally rotate and flex the baby's arm as you abduct it to elongate the side, especially the latissimus dorsi.
- Do not jerk the baby's arms. Apply traction slowly and carefully.
- Maintain both arms in external rotation.

Component Goals

- Elongation of the muscles that elevate the scapulae (upper trapezius, levator scapulae)
- Elongation of muscles on the weight-bearing side of the trunk
- Eccentric activation of the hip, trunk, and neck muscles on the weight-bearing side
- Concentric activation of the hip, trunk, and neck muscles on the unweighted side
- Sensory stimulation through the tactile, proprioceptive, visual, and vestibular systems
- Stimulation of the righting reactions through the detection of the sensory feedback
- Muscle activation for lateral righting reactions of the head and trunk

Functional Goals

- Preparation for all lateral weight shifts
- Upper-extremity preparation for reaching and protective extension
- Preparation for transitions out of sitting

8.5 Diagonal Weight Shifts: Rotation With Flexion

The goals of these facilitation techniques are for the baby to develop the ability to shift weight diagonally and use equilibrium reactions with rotation when sitting. Additional goals include detection and appropriate balance responses to changing sensory feedback, anticipation of balance requirements, and diagonal activation of trunk muscles.

Note: The entire spine and pelvis rotate over the femur; this is not rotation of the rib cage over a stable pelvis.

Baby's Position The baby sits on your legs, facing away from you (figure 8.5.1).

Therapist's Position Long-sit on the floor (figure 8.5.1), or sit on a bench with your hips flexed to 90°. You must be free to raise and lower your legs to shift the baby's weight. Therefore you cannot ring-sit.

Therapist's Hands and Movement Place your hands on the baby's trunk with your thumbs on the baby's arms (figure 8.5.1).

Raise your right leg to shift the baby's weight to the left (figure 8.5.1). At the same time, use your hands to rotate the baby's trunk to the right. Encourage the baby to reach for the right foot with both hands. Use your thumbs on the baby's arms to assist the baby to reach with both arms (figure 8.5.1).

Repeat the weight shift and rotation to the other side. Raise your left leg to shift the baby's weight to the right (figure 8.5.2). At the same time, use your hands to rotate the baby's trunk to the left.

If the baby has difficulty reaching with the far arm (figure 8.5.2, baby's right arm), slide your hand from the baby's trunk to the baby's arm, apply subtle traction to the arm, and abduct it across the baby's trunk to the foot (figures 8.5.2, 8.5.3). Your body performs the same weight shift with the baby. Failure to shift your weight will block the baby's weight shift.

While supporting the baby with one hand and your body, move your other hand to the baby's foot to bring it close to the baby's hands (figure 8.5.3). Encourage the baby to play with the foot and leg. You can incorporate this facilitation into dressing and undressing activities.

Suggestions

- It is preferable for the baby to touch and explore his or her own leg and foot. You can use this technique to apply cream to the body. Put cream on the baby's hand and have the baby spread it on the leg and foot, or put the cream on the baby's leg and have the baby reach for it with the hands.
- Use a brightly colored toy on the foot if the baby does not reach to the foot spontaneously or does not show interest in the leg or foot.

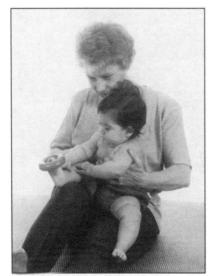

Figure 8.5.1. Diagonal weight shifts: Rotation with flexion. The therapist places both hands on the baby's trunk, with her thumbs on the baby's arms, and raises her right leg to shift the baby's weight to the left. The therapist simultaneously uses her hands to rotate the baby's trunk to the right, using her thumbs on the baby's arms to assist the baby to reach for the right foot with both hands.

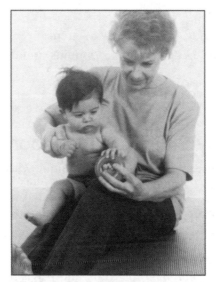

Figure 8.5.2. Weight shift and rotation to the other side. The therapist raises her left leg to shift the baby's weight to the right. Because this baby has difficulty reaching with the right arm, the therapist slides her right hand from the baby's trunk to the baby's right arm and applies subtle traction to the arm to abduct it across the baby's trunk to reach a toy at the baby's left foot.

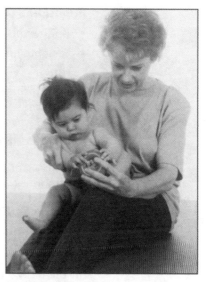

Figure 8.5.3. While supporting the baby with her right hand and body, the therapist moves her left hand to the baby's foot to bring it close to the baby's hands.

Precautions

- Initiate the rotation from the baby's trunk. Do not pull the baby's arms across the trunk.
- Apply traction carefully. If the baby resists forward reaching with the arm, reduce your pressure on the arm and return to the baby's trunk.
- Shift your weight by raising and lowering your legs.
- Your weight shifts and the raising and lowering of your legs help shift the baby's weight.
- Give the baby time to touch and explore the leg and foot.

Component Goals

- Diagonal weight shifts to facilitate trunk rotation with extension
- Upper-extremity forward reaching
- Reaching across midline
- Hand-on-body exploration
- Accommodation of the hand onto the leg and foot
- Shaping of the hands during reaching to the leg and foot
- Sensory stimulation to elicit equilibrium reactions

Functional Goals

- Body exploration to develop body awareness
- Weight shifts for dressing, such as donning and doffing socks and shoes
- Equilibrium reactions in sitting

Option: Baby Sitting on the Floor

You also can perform this facilitation technique with the baby sitting on the floor.

Therapist's Position Kneel behind the baby in a position to shift your weight with the baby.

Therapist's Hands and Movement Place both of your hands laterally on the baby's trunk and align the trunk and pelvis to neutral.

Use both hands to shift the baby's weight diagonally back to one hip (figure 8.5.4, baby's left hip). Your *guiding hand* is the hand on the baby's soon-to-be unweighted side (figure 8.5.4, therapist's right hand). Your *guiding hand* maintains the baby's neutral alignment and simultaneously shifts the baby's weight diagonally backward onto the left hip while rotating the right side of the baby's ribs and pelvis backward (figure 8.5.4).

Your *assisting hand* is the hand on the baby's soon-to-be weighted (left) side. Your *assisting hand* helps elongate the side and keep the baby's rib cage and pelvis in neutral alignment and moving as a unit. As the baby's weight shifts to the left hip, your *assisting hand* **slightly** rotates the left side of the baby's rib cage and pelvis forward (figure 8.5.4).

The baby's trunk rotation toward the unweighted leg activates the oblique abdominals, and the unweighted leg flexes, abducts, and externally rotates (figures 8.5.4 and 8.5.5).

When the baby's weight shifts, the baby may respond with an upper-extremity protective extension reaction (figure 8.5.5).

Make sure you practice the equilibrium reactions with weight shifts to both sides (figures 8.5.4 and 8.5.5). The transitions in and out of midline are a critical aspect of this facilitation.

In figure 8.5.5, the baby's weight shifts to the right hip as the therapist's left hand shifts the baby's weight diagonally backward onto the right hip while rotating the left side of the baby's ribs and pelvis backward. The therapist's right hand elongates the baby's right side and **slightly** rotates the baby's right side of the trunk forward (figure 8.5.5).

Option: Baby Sitting on a Toy

You also can practice balance reactions by diagonally tipping a flat toy on which the baby is sitting (figure 8.5.6).

Precautions

- The baby's trunk must not flex or hyperextend. It must stay aligned.
- The movement must occur on the transverse plane (rotation), not the frontal plane (lateral flexion).

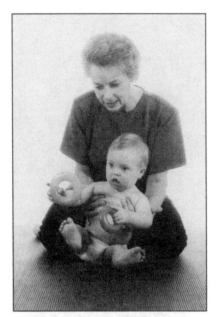

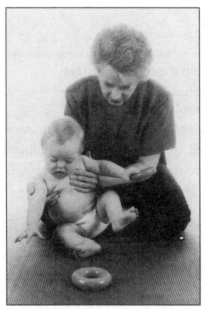

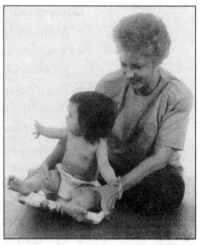

Figure 8.5.4. Option: Baby sitting on the floor. The therapist kneels behind the baby, placing both hands laterally on the baby's trunk to align the trunk and pelvis to neutral. The therapist's *guiding (right) hand* is on the baby's soon-to-be unweighted side, maintaining neutral alignment and simultaneously shifting the baby's weight diagonally backward onto the left hip while rotating the right side of the baby's ribs and pelvis backward. The therapist's *assisting (left) hand* is on the baby's soon-to-be weighted side, helping elongate the left side and keep the baby's rib cage and pelvis in neutral alignment and moving as a unit. As the baby's weight shifts to the left hip, the *assisting hand* slightly rotates the left side of the baby's rib cage and pelvis forward.

Figure 8.5.5. The therapist shifts the baby's weight diagonally backward onto the right hip while rotating the left side of the baby's ribs and pelvis backward. The baby's unweighted left leg flexes, abducts, and externally rotates. The baby also responds with a protective extension reaction with the right upper extremity.

Figure 8.5.6. Option: Baby sitting on a toy. The therapist practices balance reactions by diagonally tipping a flat toy on which the baby is sitting. The baby's weight shifts backward to the left, and the baby responds by rotating to the right.

- Do not facilitate the baby's weight laterally to one hip. Shift the baby's weight diagonally backward to one hip.
- The rib cage must not shift over the pelvis.
- The rotation must occur simultaneously in the rib cage and pelvis. The pelvis and trunk must move together as a unit over the weight-bearing femur.
- The unweighted leg must flex, abduct, and externally rotate to neutral.

Component Goals

- Mobility for spinal rotation
- Rotation with the trunk flexors working diagonally and synchronously with the trunk extensors
- Rotation of the trunk and pelvis over the femur for pelvic femoral mobility and control
- Activation of the oblique abdominals and trunk extensors
- Bilateral upper-extremity movement into shoulder flexion
- Active hip flexion, abduction, and external rotation
- Sensory input to prepare for sitting equilibrium reactions

Functional Goals

- Balance reactions to prevent a fall backward
- Balance reactions for dressing skills

8.6 Diagonal Weight Shifts: Rotation With Extension Facing Away From Therapist

The goals of this facilitation are to increase the baby's spinal, pelvic, hip, and lower-extremity mobility; to increase the baby's active head/neck rotation; and to increase the baby's experience in, and tolerance to diagonal weight shifts in the trunk, pelvis, and lower extremities.

Note: This is rotation of the entire spine, not rotation of the rib cage over the pelvis.

Baby's Position The baby straddle-sits on your leg facing away from you (figure 8.6.1).

Therapist's Position Long-sit on the floor (figure 8.6.1), or sit on a bench or ball (figure 8.6.4) with your hips flexed to 90°.

Therapist's Hands Place both of your hands on the baby's trunk, firmly holding the baby's rib cage (figure 8.6.1). If the baby's trunk is flexed, apply gentle pressure with your thumbs to extend the baby's spine. Subtly press the baby's rib cage into the pelvis while maintaining the extension, in order to connect the ribs and pelvis.

Your *guiding hand* is the hand that rotates one side of the baby's trunk forward (figure 8.6.2, therapist's left hand), and your *assisting hand* is the hand that aligns the rib cage with the pelvis and rotates the other side of the baby's trunk backward (figure 8.6.2, therapist's right hand). If the baby's trunk needs support, slide your *assisting hand* to the baby's anterior rib cage to provide that support (figure 8.6.3, therapist's left hand).

Your leg helps keep the baby's legs abducted and helps with lower-extremity dissociation as the pelvis rotates.

Movement When you have extended the baby's trunk and aligned the rib cage and pelvis, use your *guiding hand* to rotate the baby's trunk (figures 8.6.2 and 8.6.4). Rotation of the spine must facilitate rotation of the pelvis over the face-side femur. Do not rotate the rib cage over a static pelvis. This will create mobility and possibly hypermobility in the spine.

If the baby tries to retract the shoulder as the trunk rotates forward, use your index finger to hold the baby's arm forward (figure 8.6.4).

Use your *assisting hand* to guide the baby's trunk to rotate and to keep the baby's rib cage aligned with the pelvis. Do not let the baby's rib cage rotate without the pelvis, and do not let it shift laterally over the pelvis. Do not pull the baby's rib cage backward with your *assisting hand.*

When you are long-sitting, raise your leg to provide anterior support to the baby's trunk (figure 8.6.2). When the baby rotates away from your leg, slide your hand around to the baby's anterior rib cage (figure 8.6.3) to provide anterior support to the baby's trunk. Take care to not hyperextend the baby's lumbar spine when you support the anterior rib cage.

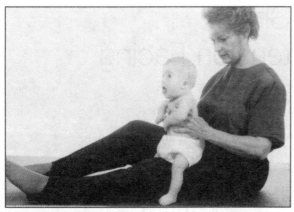

Figure 8.6.1. Diagonal weight shifts: Rotation with extension facing away from therapist. The baby straddle-sits on the therapist's leg, facing away from the therapist, who is long-sitting on the floor. The therapist places both hands on the baby's trunk, firmly holding the baby's rib cage.

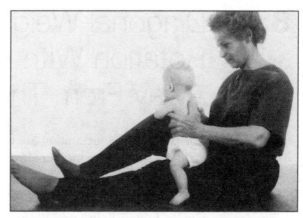

Figure 8.6.2. The therapist's *guiding (left) hand* rotates the left side of the baby's trunk forward, while the *assisting (right) hand* aligns the rib cage with the pelvis and rotates the other side of the baby's trunk backward. The therapist raises her right leg to provide anterior support to the baby's trunk.

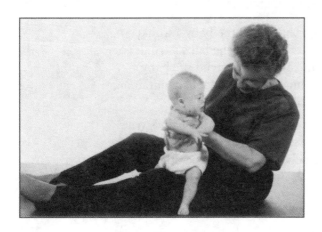

Figure 8.6.3. To support the baby's trunk when the baby rotates away from the therapist's raised leg, the therapist slides her *assisting (left) hand* around to the baby's anterior rib cage to provide anterior support to the baby's trunk and uses her *guiding (right) hand* to rotate the baby's trunk. The backward rotation of the pelvis on the baby's face side causes the baby's left femur to move toward external rotation.

Rotation of the pelvis results in a weight shift to the same side to which the face turns. Rotation of the pelvis over the femur results in hip joint rotation. The backward rotation of the pelvis on the baby's face side causes the femur to move toward external rotation (figure 8.6.3, baby's left leg; figure 8.6.4, baby's right leg). The forward rotation of the pelvis on the baby's skull side causes the femur to move toward internal rotation (figure 8.6.5, baby's right leg).

Option You may sit on a ball to perform this technique (figures 8.6.4 and 8.6.5). When you sit on the ball, you can use bouncing to increase the baby's alertness and trunk extension. Be careful to monitor the baby's ongoing responses to the bouncing. Stop bouncing if it upsets the baby.

Suggestion Use games and/or singing that encourage the baby to turn from side to side. For example, have the caregiver stand in front of the baby and move a toy from side to side to encourage the baby to turn from side to side.

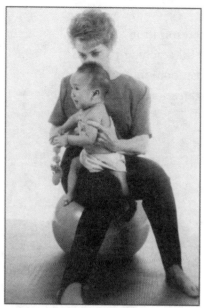 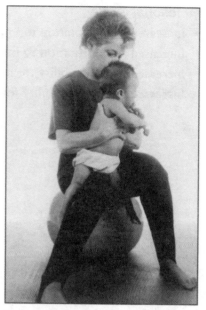

Figure 8.6.4. The therapist sits on a ball with her hips flexed to 90°, with the baby straddle-sitting on her right leg. The therapist rotates the baby's trunk with her *guiding (left) hand*. The baby tries to retract the shoulder as the trunk rotates forward, so the therapist uses her index finger to hold the baby's arm forward.

Figure 8.6.5. The forward rotation of the pelvis on the baby's skull side causes the baby's right femur to move toward internal rotation.

Precautions

- Do not push aggressively on the baby's trunk.
- Extend the thoracic spine and maintain the extension during the entire facilitation.
- Do not pull the baby's rib cage backward with your *assisting hand*.
- Do not rotate or shift the rib cage over a fixed pelvis. This dissociates the rib cage from the pelvis and leads to rib cage shifting and hypermobility between the thoracic and lumbar spines.
- Do not shift the baby's rib cage laterally over the pelvis.
- Keep both of the baby's shoulders parallel with the floor.
- Take care to not hyperextend the baby's lumbar spine when you support the anterior rib cage.

Component Goals

- Sequential spinal rotation with extension
- Pelvic-femoral (hip joint) mobility
- Lower-extremity dissociation
- Elongation of hip adductors
- Weight shift to the face side

Functional Goals

- Increased spinal rotation to improve respiration
- Increased spinal rotation to improve all reaching patterns
- Increased spinal mobility for all transitional movements
- Increased hip joint mobility for all transitional movements

8.7 Diagonal Weight Shifts: Rotation With Extension Facing Therapist

The goals of this facilitation are to increase the baby's trunk, pelvic, hip, and lower-extremity mobility; to increase upper-extremity reaching across the midline; to increase diagonal activation of trunk muscles; and to increase control of the trunk on the transverse plane.

The therapist's body provides the baby with mobility and stability, which the therapist can vary throughout the movement.

Baby's Position The baby sits on your legs facing you (figure 8.7.1).

Therapist's Position Long-sit on the floor (figure 8.7.1), or sit on a bench with your hips flexed to 90°. You must be free to raise and lower your legs to shift the baby's weight. Therefore, you cannot ring-sit.

Therapist's Hands and Movement Place your hands on the baby's rib cage, with the pads of your fingers on or near the transverse processes of the baby's spine (figure 8.7.1). Press in with the pads of your fingers and extend the baby's spine (figure 8.7.1). While maintaining the trunk extension, press down slightly to connect the rib cage to the pelvis.

If the baby has tight hip adductors, place your forearms between the baby's legs to abduct the baby's legs. If the baby has low tone with widely abducted legs, place your forearms on the lateral sides of the baby's legs to adduct the baby's legs (figure 8.7.1). The contact of your hands and arms on the baby's trunk and legs provides stability to the baby and increases the baby's confidence in the rotation and weight shift. Maintain this contact throughout the movement.

Your hands, legs, and body help facilitate the baby's rotation and weight shift. To facilitate the baby's rotation and weight shift to the left, raise your left leg and shift your weight to the right as your *guiding hand* rotates the right side of the baby's trunk forward and your *assisting hand* rotates the left side of the baby's trunk backward (figure 8.7.2).

Continue spinal rotation until the baby's pelvis rotates over the face-side femur. Make sure that the rib cage does not just rotate over a stable pelvis. This will create mobility and possibly hypermobility between the thoracic and lumbar spines.

To facilitate the baby's rotation and weight shift to the right, raise your right leg and shift your weight to the left as your *guiding hand* rotates the left side of the baby's trunk forward and your *assisting hand* rotates the right side of the baby's trunk backward (figure 8.7.3).

Your *assisting hand* maintains the elongation of the baby's side and the alignment of the ribs and pelvis and prevents lateral shifting of the rib cage (figure 8.7.2).

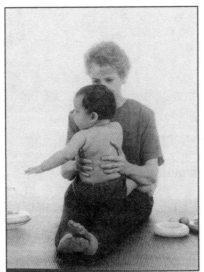

Figure 8.7.1. Diagonal weight shifts: Rotation with extension facing therapist. The therapist long-sits on the floor with the baby sitting on her legs, facing her. The therapist places both hands on the baby's rib cage, with the pads of the fingers on or near the transverse processes of the baby's spine. She presses in with the pads of her fingers, extending the baby's spine and pressing down slightly to connect the rib cage to the pelvis. The therapist places her forearms on the lateral side of the baby's legs to adduct them.

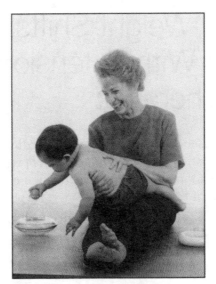

Figure 8.7.2. To facilitate the baby's rotation and weight shift to the left, the therapist raises her left leg and shifts her weight to the right as her *guiding hand* rotates the right side of the baby's trunk forward. Her *assisting hand* rotates the left side of the baby's trunk backward, maintaining the elongation of the baby's side and the alignment of the ribs and pelvis and preventing lateral shifting of the rib cage.

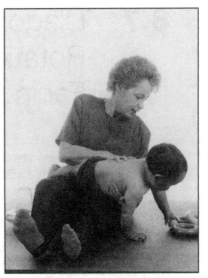

Figure 8.7.3. To facilitate the baby's rotation and weight shift to the right, the therapist raises her right leg and shifts her weight to the left as her *guiding hand* rotates the left side of the baby's trunk forward and her *assisting hand* rotates the right side of the baby's trunk backward. The therapist places one of the baby's hands on the floor for extended-arm weight bearing while the baby reaches across the trunk with the other arm.

If the baby has sufficient trunk and hip mobility, place one of the baby's hands on the floor for extended-arm weight bearing while the baby reaches across the trunk with the other arm (figure 8.7.3). When the baby maintains the extended-arm weight-bearing position while actively reaching across the body with the other arm, the baby's shoulder girdle muscles are very dynamic.

Make sure you rotate the baby to both sides.

Suggestion Use toys to engage the baby's active participation in the rotation. The baby can reach for a toy on one side, pick it up, and place it on the other side. If the baby has difficulty with upper-extremity reaching, use games and/or singing that encourage the baby to turn from side to side. For example, you may have the caregiver stand behind you and play peek-a-boo from side to side to encourage the baby to turn from side to side.

Precautions

- Never force the baby to rotate.
- Keep the baby's trunk extended throughout the facilitation.

- Take care to maintain rib cage-pelvic alignment.
- Rotate the pelvis with the rest of the trunk. Do not rotate the ribs over a fixed pelvis.
- Keep your forearms in contact with the baby's legs throughout the rotation. This provides a point of stability for the baby.

Component Goals

- Sequential spinal rotation
- Pelvic-femoral (hip joint) mobility
- Lower-extremity dissociation
- Elongation of hip adductors
- Active hip extension with abduction (unweighted leg) for balance in the trunk
- Active control in the leg to assist with balance in the trunk
- Activation of the oblique abdominals when returning to sit
- Shoulder flexion with adduction
- Activation of shoulder-girdle muscles

Functional Goals

- Postural control for sitting while using the upper extremities
- Mobility and control for upper-extremity reaching across the body
- Trunk mobility for transitions from sitting to prone or sitting to quadruped
- Lower-extremity mobility for walking

9. Sitting on Lap Sequences

9.1 Rotation to Stand With Extension: Facing Therapist

The goal of this facilitation is to teach the baby to rise to unilateral stance from sitting. Additional goals are to sequence and increase the baby's trunk, pelvic, hip, and lower-extremity mobility; to increase lower-extremity dissociation; and to increase the baby's trunk and lower-extremity control in unilateral stance. Unilateral standing with lower-extremity dissociation helps prepare the legs for forward walking.

Baby's Position The baby straddle-sits on your leg, facing you (figure 9.1.1).

Therapist's Position Long-sit on the floor (figure 9.1.1). You must be free to raise and lower your legs to assist the baby. Therefore, you cannot ring-sit.

Therapist's Hands and Movement

Initiation
Place your hands on the baby's rib cage, with the pads of your fingers on or near the transverse processes of the baby's spine (figure 9.1.1). Press in with the pads of your fingers and extend the baby's spine. While maintaining the trunk extension, press down slightly to connect the rib cage to the pelvis.

Use both hands to rotate the baby's trunk so the weight shifts to one leg (figure 9.1.2). Your *guiding hand* rotates the right side of the baby's trunk forward (figure 9.1.2, therapist's left hand) while your *assisting hand* maintains the alignment of the baby's rib cage and pelvis, prevents lateral shifting of the rib cage, and rotates the left side of the baby's trunk backward (figure 9.1.2, therapist's right hand).

Continue spinal rotation until the baby's pelvis rotates over the face-side femur and the baby's weight shifts to that leg. Make sure the rib cage does not rotate over a stable pelvis. This will create mobility and possibly hypermobility between the thoracic and lumbar spines.

To Stand
When the baby's weight has shifted to the face-side leg, stabilize the baby's trunk with your *assisting hand* and move your *guiding hand* to the baby's back leg, placing it close to the baby's knee (figure 9.1.3).

Use both of your hands to transition the baby to standing. Use your *assisting hand* to support the baby's trunk, maintain trunk extension, and lift the baby's weight diagonally forward and up over one leg. Use your *guiding hand* to rotate the baby's back femur internally to neutral,

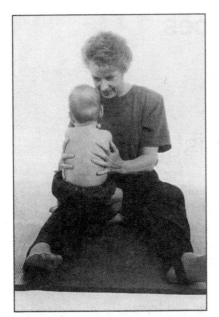

Figure 9.1.1. Rotation to stand with extension: Facing therapist. Initiation. The baby straddle-sits on the therapist's leg, facing her. The therapist places both hands on the baby's rib cage, with the pads of the fingers on or near the transverse processes of the baby's spine. She presses in with the pads of her fingers to extend the baby's spine and presses down slightly to connect the rib cage to the pelvis.

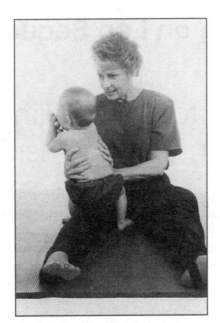

Figure 9.1.2. The therapist uses both hands to facilitate the baby's rotation and weight shift to the left. Her *guiding hand* rotates the right side of the baby's trunk forward. Her *assisting hand* rotates the left side of the baby's trunk backward, maintaining the alignment of the ribs and pelvis and preventing lateral shifting of the rib cage.

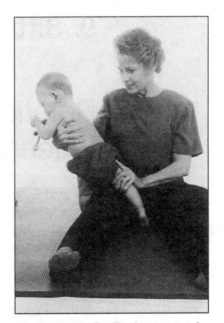

Figure 9.1.3. Facilitation to stand. When the baby's weight has shifted to the face-side leg, the therapist stabilizes the baby's trunk with her *assisting hand* and moves her *guiding hand* to the baby's back (right) leg, placing it close to the baby's knee. The therapist uses both hands to shift the baby's weight: she supports the baby's trunk, maintains trunk extension, and lifts the baby's weight diagonally forward and up over the left leg with her *assisting hand*; the *guiding hand* simultaneously rotates the baby's right femur internally to neutral, extends the baby's right hip and knee, and compresses the femur into the pelvis to shift the baby's weight forward and up onto the face-side (left) leg.

at the same time extending the baby's back hip and knee and compressing the femur into the pelvis so you shift the baby's weight forward and up onto the face-side leg (figure 9.1.3).

When the baby rises to stand, the forward leg is in a position similar to the midstance position of the gait cycle. The back leg is in a position similar to the initial swing position of the gait cycle.

Backward Weight Shift

With the baby's weight on the forward leg, continue to support and extend the baby's trunk with your *assisting hand* (figure 9.1.4). With your *guiding hand*, maintain the baby's hip in neutral rotation and the hip and knee in extension. Place the baby's toes on the floor (figure

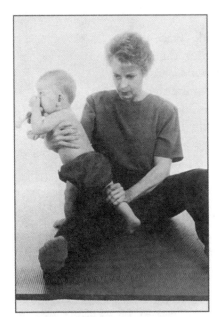

Figure 9.1.4. Backward weight shift. The therapist continues to support and extend the baby's trunk with her *assisting hand* while her *guiding hand* maintains the baby's right hip and knee in extension and continues to rotate the baby's femur internally until it is in neutral rotation. The therapist then places the toes of the baby's right foot on the floor.

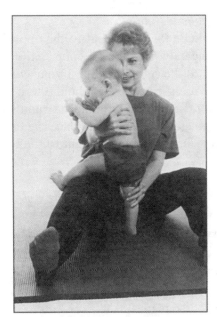

Figure 9.1.5. Once the baby's toes are on the floor, the therapist uses her *guiding hand* to keep the right hip and knee extended while pressing the leg back and down until the baby's heel is on the floor. At the same time, the therapist uses her *assisting hand* to guide the baby's trunk backward over the leg, raising her leg to support the baby's front (left) leg as the baby's weight shifts backward.

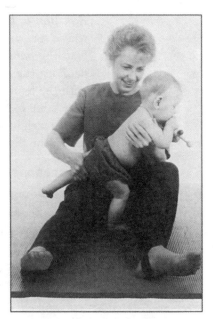

Figure 9.1.6. Rotation to the opposite side. The therapist's *assisting (left) hand* is on the baby's trunk and her *guiding (right) hand* is on the baby's back (left) leg. The thumb of the *guiding hand* is parallel with the femur and presses it up toward the hip to help facilitate the baby's hip extension.

9.1.4, baby's right foot). This lower-extremity position is similar to the position of terminal stance or push-off in the gait cycle.

Once the baby's toes are on the floor, use your *assisting hand* to guide the baby's trunk backward over the leg (figure 9.1.5, baby's right leg). At the same time, use your *guiding hand* to keep the hip and knee extended while you press the leg back and down until the baby's heel is on the floor (figure 9.1.5). This elongates the baby's toe flexors and gastrocnemius/soleus muscles.

As the baby's weight shifts backward, raise your leg so that it supports the baby's front leg (figure 9.1.5, baby's left leg). This position elongates the baby's hamstring muscles.

When the baby's weight shifts backward, the back leg is in a position similar to the midstance phase of the gait cycle. The front leg is in a position similar to the swing phase of gait. Alternate the baby between bearing weight on the front leg (figure 9.1.4) and bearing weight on the back leg (figure 9.1.5) so the baby can experience the various components and phases of the gait cycle.

Rotation to the Opposite Side

Make sure you facilitate the movement to the opposite side. Place your *assisting hand* on the baby's trunk and your *guiding hand* on the baby's back leg (figure 9.1.6). Place the thumb of your *guiding hand* parallel with the femur and press it up toward the hip to help facilitate the baby's hip extension (figure 9.1.6, therapist's right hand). Once the baby's weight is stable on the front leg, place the toes of the baby's back leg on the floor and shift the baby's weight to the back leg.

Precautions

- Never force the baby to rotate.
- Keep the baby's trunk extended throughout the facilitation technique.
- Take care to maintain rib cage-pelvic alignment.
- Shift the baby's weight to the face-side leg before attempting to bring the baby to stand.
- Once the baby is in standing, the baby's pelvis must be in neutral alignment on all three planes.
- Support the baby's trunk throughout the movement.
- Keep the baby's back hip and knee extended.
- Slowly rotate the baby's back hip internally to neutral. Internal rotation of the femur produces forward rotation of the pelvis and assists with the baby's trunk rotation.
- Slowly elongate the baby's toe flexors and gastrocnemius/soleus muscles during the backward weight shift.
- Carefully elongate the baby's hamstrings. Do not force the elongation.

Component Goals

- Sequential spinal and pelvic rotation
- Spinal rotation with extension
- Pelvic-femoral (hip joint) mobility
- Lower-extremity dissociation
- Active hip and knee extension
- Elongation of hip adductors
- Elongation of the hamstrings
- Elongation of toe flexors and gastrocnemius/soleus muscles

Functional Goals

- Preparation for independent rising to stand from sitting
- Lower-extremity dissociation in preparation for walking
- Preparation for midstance, swing, and push-off phases of the gait cycle
- Preparation for weight transfer in the feet during the stance phases of the gait cycle

9.2 Rotation to Stand With Extension: Facing Away From Therapist

The goal of this facilitation is to teach the baby to rise to unilateral stance from sitting. Additional goals are to sequence and increase the baby's trunk, pelvic, hip, and lower-extremity mobility; to increase lower-extremity dissociation; and to increase the baby's trunk and lower-extremity control in unilateral stance. Unilateral standing with lower-extremity dissociation helps prepare the legs for forward walking.

This technique is the same as the previous technique except that the baby initiates the movement facing away from the therapist.

Baby's Position The baby straddle-sits on your leg, facing away from you (figure 9.2.1).

Therapist's Position Long-sit on the floor (figure 9.2.1). You must be free to raise and lower your legs to assist the baby with the movement. Therefore you cannot ring-sit.

Therapist's Hands and Movement Place your *assisting hand* on the baby's anterior rib cage and extend the baby's trunk (figure 9.2.1, therapist's right hand). Use your *guiding hand* to align the baby's pelvis and femurs so the baby's hips flex to 90° (figure 9.2.1, therapist's left hand). Then place your *guiding hand* on the baby's leg near the knee with your fingers around the baby's femur and your thumb parallel to the femur and, if possible, across the baby's hip joint (figure 9.2.2).

Use your *assisting hand* to rotate the baby's trunk, being careful to rotate the pelvis with the rib cage. If the baby tries to retract the shoulder as the trunk rotates forward, slide your *assisting hand* around the baby's trunk and hold the baby's arm forward during the rotation (figure 9.2.2). Support the baby's trunk with the arm of your *assisting hand*.

Continue trunk rotation until the baby's pelvis rotates over the face-side femur and the baby's weight shifts to that leg. As the baby's weight shifts to the face-side leg, use your *assisting hand* to maintain trunk extension and support the baby's trunk and flexed arms while bringing the baby's weight diagonally forward and up over the forward leg (figure 9.2.2). You may raise your free leg to give the baby a surface for which to reach.

As the baby rises to stand, use your *guiding hand* to internally rotate the baby's back femur slightly, extend the baby's back hip and knee, and compress the femur into the pelvis to help shift the baby's weight forward and up onto the face-side leg (figure 9.2.2).

When the baby rises to stand, the forward leg is in a position similar to the midstance position of the gait cycle. The back leg is in a position similar to the initial swing position of the gait cycle.

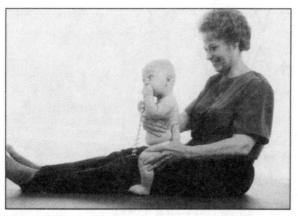

Figure 9.2.1. Rotation to stand with extension: Facing away from therapist. The baby straddle-sits on the therapist's leg, facing away from her. The therapist uses her *assisting (right) hand* on the baby's anterior rib cage to extend the baby's trunk. The *guiding (left) hand* aligns the baby's pelvis and femurs so the baby's hips flex to 90°.

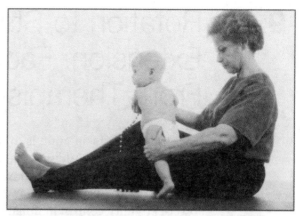

Figure 9.2.2. Facilitation to stand. As the baby's weight shifts to the face-side leg, the therapist uses her *assisting hand* to maintain trunk extension and hold the flexed arms while bringing the baby's weight diagonally forward and up over the forward leg. The therapist raises her free leg to give the baby a surface for which to reach. The therapist's *guiding hand* internally rotates the baby's back femur slightly, extends the baby's back hip and knee, and compresses the femur into the pelvis to help shift the baby's weight forward and up onto the face-side leg.

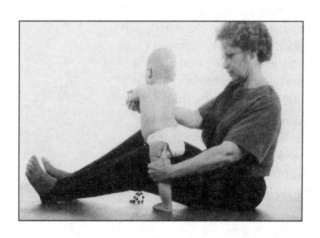

Figure 9.2.3. Backward weight shift. The therapist uses her *guiding hand* to place the toes of the baby's back (left) foot on the floor, keep the hip and knee extended, and press the leg down and back until the baby's heel is on the floor. The therapist uses her *assisting hand* to guide the baby's trunk backward over the left leg. As the baby's weight shifts backward, the therapist raises her leg to support the baby's front leg and to help extend the baby's back leg.

Backward Weight Shift

To shift the baby's weight to the back leg, maintain the baby's hip and knee in extension with neutral hip rotation and place the toes of the baby's back foot on the floor with your *guiding hand*. Continue to extend and support the baby's trunk and arms with your *assisting hand*.

Once the baby's toes are on the floor, use your *assisting hand* to guide the baby's trunk backward over the leg. At the same time, use your *guiding hand* to keep the hip and knee extended while you press the leg down and back until the baby's heel is on the floor (figure 9.2.3).

As the baby's weight shifts to the back foot, raise your leg to support the baby's front leg and help extend the baby's back leg (figure 9.2.3). This elongates the hamstring muscles on the front leg.

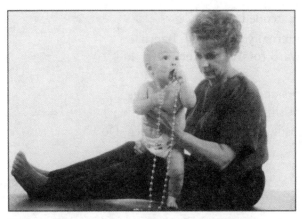

Figure 9.2.4. Rotation to the opposite side. The therapist places her *assisting hand* on the baby's trunk and her *guiding hand* on the baby's back leg, rotates the baby's trunk so the weight shifts to the face-side leg, then uses both hands to transition the baby to stand.

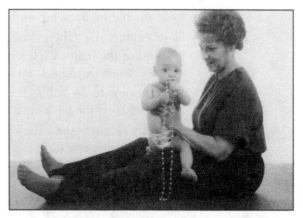

Figure 9.2.5. The therapist continues to support and extend the baby's trunk with her *assisting hand* and maintains the baby's hip in neutral rotation and the hip and knee in extension with her *guiding hand*. She then shifts the baby's weight backward to the back leg, raising her leg to support the baby's front leg.

When the baby's weight shifts backward, the back leg is in a position similar to the midstance phase of the gait cycle. The front leg is in a position similar to the swing phase of gait. Alternate the baby between bearing weight on the front leg (figure 9.2.2) and bearing weight on the back leg (figure 9.2.3) so the baby can experience the various components and phases of the gait cycle.

Rotation to the Opposite Side
Make sure you facilitate the movement to the opposite sides (figures 9.2.4 and 9.2.5).

Place your *assisting hand* on the baby's trunk and your *guiding hand* on the baby's back leg. Rotate the baby's trunk so the weight shifts to the face-side leg. Use both hands to transition the baby to stand (figure 9.2.4).

Continue to support and extend the baby's trunk with your *assisting hand* and maintain the baby's hip in neutral rotation and the hip and knee in extension with your *guiding hand* as you shift the baby's weight backward to the back leg. Raise your leg to support the baby's front leg (figure 9.2.5).

Help the baby alternately transition between bearing weight on the front leg (figure 9.2.4) and the back leg (figure 9.2.5). The weight shifts help prepare the baby's legs and trunk for forward walking.

Precautions
- Never force the baby to rotate.
- Keep the baby's trunk extended.
- Take care to maintain rib cage-pelvic alignment.
- Flex both arms forward.
- Shift the baby's weight to the face-side leg before attempting to bring the baby to stand.
- Support the baby's trunk throughout the movement.

- Keep the baby's back hip and knee extended.
- Slowly rotate the baby's back hip internally to neutral. Internal rotation of the femur produces forward rotation of the pelvis and assists the baby's trunk rotation.
- Slowly elongate the baby's toe flexors and gastrocnemius/soleus muscles during the backward weight shift.
- Carefully elongate the baby's hamstrings on the baby's front leg. Do not force the elongation.

Component Goals
- Sequential spinal and pelvic rotation
- Spinal rotation with extension
- Pelvic-femoral (hip joint) mobility
- Lower-extremity dissociation
- Active hip and knee extension
- Elongation of hip adductors
- Elongation of the hamstrings
- Elongation of toe flexors and gastrocnemius/soleus muscles

Functional Goals
- Preparation for independent rising to stand from sitting
- Lower-extremity dissociation in preparation for walking
- Preparation for midstance and push-off phases of the gait cycle
- Preparation for weight transfer in the feet during the stance phases of the gait cycle

9.3   Rotation to Stand at a Table

The goal of this facilitation is to teach the baby to rise to unilateral stance from sitting while using the upper extremities for support. Additional goals are to sequence and increase the baby's trunk, pelvic, hip, and lower-extremity mobility; to increase lower-extremity dissociation; to increase the baby's trunk and lower-extremity control in rising to stand; and to increase upper-extremity reaching and weight bearing. Unilateral standing with lower-extremity dissociation helps prepare the legs for forward walking.

This technique is similar to the previous technique except that the baby is rising to stand at a table and is reaching and supporting on the upper extremities.

Baby's Position   The baby straddle-sits on your leg, facing away from you (figure 9.3.1).

Therapist's Position   Long-sit on the floor (figure 9.3.1). You must be free to raise and lower your legs to assist the baby. Therefore, you cannot ring-sit.

Therapist's Hands and Movement   Place your hands on the baby's rib cage and extend the baby's trunk while keeping the baby's hips flexed.

Use both hands to rotate the baby's trunk so that the weight shifts to one leg. Your *guiding hand* rotates the baby's trunk forward while your *assisting hand* maintains the alignment between the baby's rib cage and pelvis. If the baby retracts the back shoulder girdle, place your *guiding hand* on the baby's arm with your forearm on the baby's trunk (figure 9.3.1). Use your *guiding-hand forearm* to assist with rotation of the baby's trunk.

Continue spinal rotation until the baby's pelvis rotates over the face-side femur, the baby's weight shifts to that leg, and the baby's hands are on the table (figure 9.3.1).

When the baby's weight shifts to the face-side leg and the baby's hands are stable on the table, move your *guiding hand* to the baby's back leg

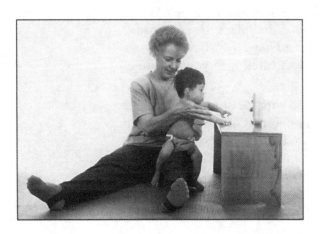

Figure 9.3.1. Rotation to stand at a table. The baby straddle-sits on the therapist's leg, facing away from her. The therapist places both hands on the baby's rib cage and extends the baby's trunk while keeping the baby's hips flexed. The therapist places her right forearm on the baby's trunk and her *guiding hand* on the baby's right arm to prevent retraction of the shoulder girdle. She then rotates the baby's trunk until the baby's pelvis rotates over the face-side (left) femur, the baby's weight shifts to that leg, and the baby's hands are on the table.

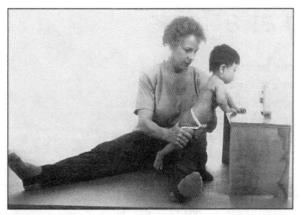

Figure 9.3.2. Facilitation to stand. The therapist uses both hands to rotate the baby to stand. She moves her *guiding hand* to the baby's back leg near the knee with her thumb parallel to the femur to rotate the femur internally to neutral, to extend the baby's back hip and knee, and to compress the femur into the pelvis so as to shift the baby's weight forward and up onto the face-side leg and hands. The *assisting hand* supports the baby's trunk, maintains trunk extension, and lifts the baby's weight diagonally forward and up over one leg and both hands.

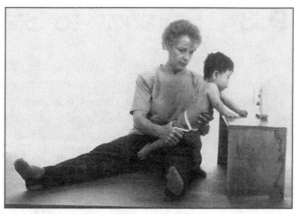

Figure 9.3.3. For a baby with low tone and/or hypermobility in the lower trunk, the therapist slides her *assisting hand* down to support and align the rib cage and lower trunk.

near the knee with your thumb parallel to the femur (figure 9.3.2). Keep your *assisting hand* on the baby's trunk.

Use both of your hands to transition the baby to stand. Use your *assisting hand* to support the baby's trunk, maintain trunk extension, and lift the baby's weight diagonally forward and up over one leg and both hands. Use your *guiding hand* to rotate the baby's back femur internally to neutral, at the same time extending the baby's back hip and knee and compressing the femur into the pelvis so that you shift the baby's weight forward and up onto the face-side leg and hands (figures 9.3.2 and 9.3.3).

If the baby has low tone and/or hypermobility in the lower trunk, slide your *assisting hand* down to support and align the rib cage and lower trunk (figure 9.3.3).

Backward Weight Shift
To shift the baby's weight to the back leg, maintain the baby's hip and knee in extension with neutral hip rotation and place the toes of the baby's back foot on the floor with your *guiding hand* (figure 9.3.4). Continue to extend and support the baby's trunk with your *assisting hand* (figure 9.3.4).

Once the baby's toes are on the floor, use your *assisting hand* to guide the baby's trunk backward over the leg (figure 9.3.5). At the same time, use your *guiding hand* to keep the hip and knee extended while you press the leg back and down until the baby's heel is on the floor (figure 9.3.5). This elongates the baby's toe flexors and gastrocnemius/soleus muscles.

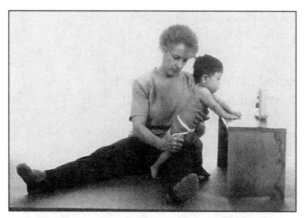

Figure 9.3.4. Backward weight shift. The therapist continues to extend and support the baby's trunk with her *assisting hand* while the *guiding hand* maintains the baby's hip and knee in extension, internally rotates the baby's femur to neutral rotation, and places the baby's toes on the floor.

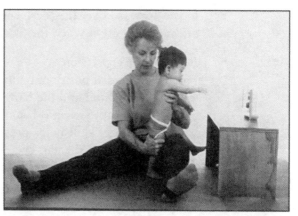

Figure 9.3.5. Once the baby's toes are on the floor, the therapist uses her *guiding hand* to keep the hip and knee extended while she presses the leg down and back until the baby's heel is on the floor. The therapist simultaneously uses her *assisting hand* to guide the baby's trunk backward over the leg. As the baby's weight shifts backward, the therapist raises her leg to help extend the baby's back leg and support the baby's front leg.

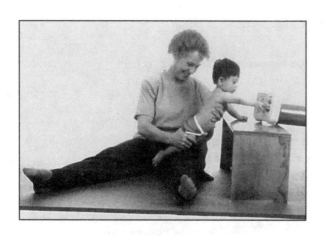

Figure 9.3.6. Maintaining control of the baby's trunk with the *assisting hand* and the baby's back leg with the *guiding hand*, the therapist shifts the baby's weight to the forward leg and upper extremities The weight shift helps prepare the baby's legs and trunk for forward walking. The baby bears weight on one arm while reaching for a toy with the other arm.

As the baby's weight shifts backward, raise your leg so that it supports the baby's front leg (figure 9.3.5). This position elongates the baby's hamstring muscles.

Alternate Between Bearing Weight on the Back Leg and the Front Leg

Forward Weight Shift

While maintaining control of the baby's trunk with your *assisting hand* and the baby's back leg with your *guiding hand*, shift the baby's weight to the forward leg and upper extremities (figure 9.3.6). When the weight shifts forward, the baby bears weight on one arm and reaches for the toy with the other arm.

The forward weight shift helps prepare the baby's legs and trunk for forward walking. The back leg moves from a midstance position when the foot is flat to a terminal-stance, or push-off, position as the weight moves forward over the toes. The front leg moves from swing to a midstance position when the front foot is flat on the floor.

Backward Weight Shift

From the forward position, maintain control of the baby's trunk with your *assisting hand* and the baby's back leg with your *guiding hand*, and shift the baby's weight backward to the back leg (figure 9.3.5). The backward weight shift helps prepare the baby's back leg and trunk for the stance phase of the gait cycle and elongates the hamstrings of the baby's front leg for the swing phase of the gait cycle.

Alternate the baby between the forward weight shift and the backward weight shift.

Reverse Sides

Make sure you facilitate the movement to the opposite side.

Suggestion Use a toy that interests and motivates the baby to stand and reach.

Precautions

- Never force the baby to rotate.
- Keep the baby's trunk extended.
- Take care to maintain rib cage-pelvic alignment.
- Flex both arms forward.
- Shift the baby's weight to the face-side leg before attempting to bring the baby to stand.
- Support the baby's trunk throughout the movement.
- Keep the baby's back hip and knee extended.
- Slowly rotate the baby's back hip internally to neutral. Internal rotation of the femur produces forward rotation of the pelvis and assists with the baby's trunk rotation.
- Slowly elongate the baby's toe flexors and gastrocnemius/soleus muscles during the backward weight shift.
- Carefully elongate the baby's hamstrings. Do not force the elongation.

Component Goals

- Sequential spinal and pelvic rotation
- Spinal rotation with extension
- Pelvic-femoral (hip joint) mobility
- Lower-extremity dissociation
- Active hip and knee extension
- Elongation of hip adductors
- Elongation of the hamstrings
- Elongation of toe flexors and gastrocnemius/soleus muscles
- Upper-extremity weight bearing and reaching

Functional Goals

- Preparation for independent rising to stand from sitting
- Lower-extremity dissociation in preparation for walking
- Preparation for transition between midstance and push-off phases of the gait cycle
- Preparation for the transition between swing and midstance phases of the gait cycle
- Preparation for weight transfer in the feet during the stance phases of the gait cycle

9.4 Rotation to Half-Kneeling

The goals of this facilitation are to increase the baby's trunk, hip, and lower-extremity mobility and control for half-kneeling and to increase the baby's balance in half-kneeling. The ultimate functional goal is for the baby to move independently into and out of half-kneeling.

Baby's Position The baby sits straddling your leg, with hips and knees at 90° (figures 9.4.1 and 9.4.4). The baby's knees should not flex more than 90°.

Your leg must be approximately the same height as the baby's femur. If your leg is too big, the baby will not be able to half-kneel around it. If your leg is too small, it will not provide the needed support for the baby's lower-extremity dissociation. Use a bolster if your leg is not the appropriate height for the baby.

Therapist's Position Long-sit on the floor (figure 9.4.1). You must be free to raise and lower your legs to assist the baby with the movement. Therefore, you cannot ring-sit.

Therapist's Hands and Movement Place your hands on the baby's rib cage and extend the baby's trunk while keeping the baby's hips flexed (figure 9.4.1).

Once you have extended the baby's trunk, place your *assisting hand* under the baby's near arm and hold the baby's far arm (figures 9.4.2 and 9.4.4). Support the baby's trunk with the arm of your *assisting hand*. Place your *guiding hand* on the baby's back leg with your fingers on the femur and the tibia and your thumb parallel to the femur (figures 9.4.2 and 9.4.5).

Use your forearm and *assisting hand* to rotate the baby's trunk until the baby's pelvis rotates over the face-side femur and the baby's weight shifts to that leg (figure 9.4.2). Make sure that the rib cage does not rotate over a stable pelvis. Do not try to rotate the baby's trunk by just pulling the baby's arm. You may create excessive scapular mobility rather that trunk rotation.

Use your *guiding hand* to rotate the baby's hip internally to neutral and extend it while flexing the knee and placing it on the floor (figures 9.4.2, 9.4.3, 9.4.5, and 9.4.6). The baby's forward leg remains in flexion by weight bearing on your leg (figure 9.4.3).

Once you have placed the baby's knee on the floor in a weight-bearing position, use your thumb to extend the baby's hip (figures 9.4.3 and 9.4.6). Your *assisting hand* on the baby's trunk shifts the baby's weight backward onto the extended hip (figure 9.4.3).

When you have aligned the baby's trunk over the extended hip and the baby is stable in the half-kneel position, move your *guiding hand* to the baby's pelvis. Spread your fingers and stabilize the baby's entire pelvis and weight-bearing leg (figure 9.4.7). Raise your opposite leg to provide the baby a stable place to rest the upper extremities (figure 9.4.7).

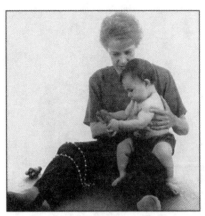

Figure 9.4.1. Rotation to half-kneeling. The baby sits straddling the therapist's leg with hips and knees at 90°. The therapist places both hands on the baby's rib cage and extends the baby's trunk while keeping the baby's hips flexed.

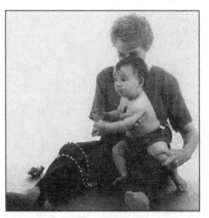

Figure 9.4.2. The therapist places her *assisting hand* under the baby's near-arm, supports the baby's trunk with her forearm, holds the baby's far arm, then rotates the baby's trunk with her forearm and *assisting hand*. She places her *guiding hand* on the baby's back leg and internally rotates and extends the baby's hip to neutral while flexing the knee.

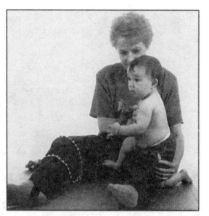

Figure 9.4.3. The therapist uses her *guiding hand* to internally rotate and extend the baby's hip to neutral while flexing the knee and placing it on the floor in a weight-bearing position, using her thumb to extend the baby's hip. The therapist's *assisting hand* on the baby's trunk shifts the baby's weight back onto the extended hip. The baby's forward leg remains in flexion by weight bearing on the therapist's leg.

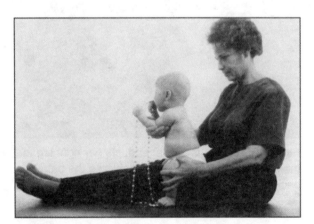

Figure 9.4.4. Back view of the facilitation. Note the therapist's *assisting hand* on the baby's left arm to prevent retraction of the left shoulder girdle. The therapist places her *guiding hand* on the baby's leg in preparation for the transition.

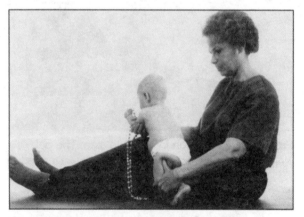

Figure 9.4.5. Back view of the facilitation. The therapist uses her *guiding hand* to internally rotate and extend the baby's hip to neutral while flexing the knee. The therapist's *assisting hand* holds the baby's arm and assists with the trunk rotation. The therapist has raised her right leg to give the baby a target for which to reach.

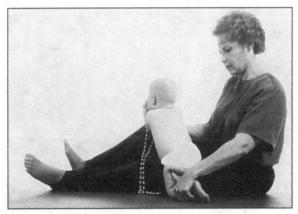

Figure 9.4.6. Back view of the facilitation. The therapist's *guiding hand* continues to extend and rotate the baby's hip internally to neutral while flexing the knee and placing it on the floor in a weight-bearing position. She uses her thumb to extend the baby's hip.

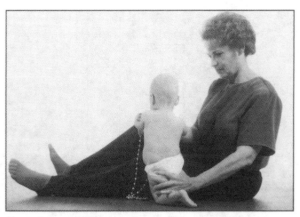

Figure 9.4.7. Once the therapist has aligned the baby's trunk over the extended hip and the baby is stable in the half-kneel position, the therapist moves her *guiding hand* and spreads her fingers to stabilize the baby's entire pelvis and weight-bearing leg. She raises her opposite leg to provide the baby a stable place to rest the upper extremities.

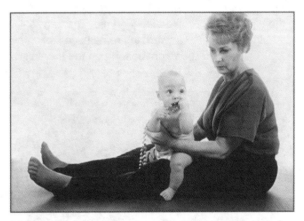

Figure 9.4.8. Rotation to opposite side. The baby's weight-bearing leg is between the therapist's legs.

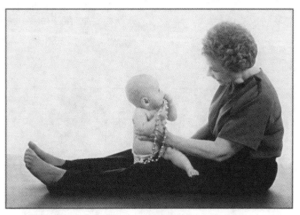

Figure 9.4.9. The therapist adducts her right leg to the baby's back hip and thus stabilizes the baby's back hip in extension.

Return to Sitting

Return the baby to sitting on your leg by rotating the baby's trunk back to its original erect position. Control the baby's back hip with your *guiding hand* as your *assisting hand* rotates the baby's trunk back.

Rotation to Opposite Side

Make sure you rotate the baby to the opposite side (figures 9.4.8 and 9.4.9). When the baby's weight-bearing leg is between your legs (figure 9.4.8), you can adduct your leg to the baby's back hip and thus stabilize the baby's back hip in extension (figure 9.4.9).

Precautions

- Never force the baby to rotate.
- Keep the baby's trunk extended throughout the facilitation technique.

- Internally rotate the back hip to neutral. If the hip remains externally rotated, the hip cannot extend and you will not be able to shift the baby's weight onto the back leg.
- Align the trunk over the extended hip. You may have to shift the baby's trunk laterally when you shift it posteriorly.
- Keep the baby's arms forward.

Component Goals
- Trunk and pelvic rotation over the femur
- Lower-extremity dissociation
- Pelvic-femoral (hip joint) mobility on all three planes
- Hip extension, internal rotation to neutral, and adduction to neutral on the back leg
- Elongation of hip flexors, external rotators, and abductors
- Elongation of knee extensors on the back leg
- Hip flexion, external rotation to neutral, and abduction to neutral on the front leg
- Elongation of hip extensors, internal rotators, and adductors on the front leg
- Elongation of knee extensors on the front leg
- Elongation of ankle dorsiflexors on the back leg and plantar flexors on the front leg

Functional Goals
- Lower-extremity mobility, preparation for the transition from sitting to half-kneeling and kneeling to half-kneeling
- Movement of the trunk and pelvis over the lower extremities in preparation for use in higher-level transitions

10. Sitting on Ball

10.1 Trunk-Pelvic-Hip Neutral Alignment and Sensory Preparation

The goals of this facilitation are to achieve trunk-pelvic-hip alignment in sitting, and to activate the baby through the sensory stimulation of bouncing.

Therapists can use the sensory preparation of bouncing to alert the baby, calm the baby, and/or engage and play with the baby.

Baby's Position The baby sits on the ball facing you, with the hips in the center of the ball.

Therapist's Position Kneel in front of the baby, at or below eye level. You must be in a position that permits you to shift your weight with the baby.

Therapist's Hands and Movement Place your hands on the baby's trunk and rest your arms on the ball and on the lateral aspects of the baby's femurs (figure 10.1.1). The contact of your arms on the baby's legs and the ball provides security to the baby and stability to the ball. You also may contact the ball with your legs for more control of the ball's movements.

If the baby's trunk flexes and the neck hyperextends (figure 10.1.1), correct this problem before going further with the facilitation technique. Use the pads of your fingers to press in along the baby's spine and extend the baby's spine (figure 10.1.2). Simultaneously bring the baby's trunk forward to align the trunk with the pelvis so the shoulders are directly over the hips (figure 10.1.2). When you have aligned the baby's trunk and pelvis, give downward pressure from the trunk into the pelvis to reinforce the base of support.

Once the baby's pelvis and trunk are in neutral alignment, maintain the baby's stability on the ball and bounce the baby up and down at various speeds. Carefully observe the baby's responses to the bouncing and modify, continue, or stop the bouncing according to those responses. If the baby tolerates the bouncing and becomes more alert, calm, and/or engaged, you can roll the ball so the baby sits with different postures on the ball. The changes in postures bring about activation of different muscles. See facilitation 10.2, Trunk-Pelvic-Hip Neutral Alignment: Weight Shifts.

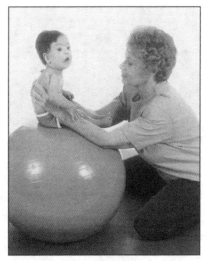 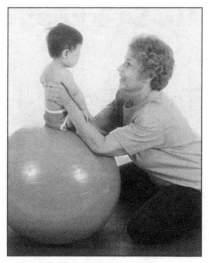

Figure 10.1.1. Trunk-pelvic-hip neutral alignment and sensory preparation. The therapist seats the baby on the ball facing her, with the baby's hips in the center of the ball. The therapist places her hands on the baby's trunk, resting her arms on the ball and on the lateral aspects of the baby's femurs. The therapist must correct the baby's problems of trunk flexion and neck hyperextension before going further with the facilitation technique.

Figure 10.1.2. The therapist corrects the baby's trunk flexion and neck hyperextension by pressing in along the baby's spine with the pads of her fingers and extending the spine. The therapist simultaneously brings the baby's trunk forward to align the trunk with the pelvis so the shoulders are directly over the hips.

Precautions

- Do not bounce the baby up and down if the trunk and pelvis are not in neutral alignment.
- Do not continue the bouncing if the baby has an adverse response such as distressed facial expressions, crying, or changes in color, vocalizations, or respiration.

Component Goals

- Neutral alignment of the pelvis over the femurs
- Neutral alignment of the spine and head over the pelvis
- Vestibular stimulation
- Proprioceptive stimulation

Functional Goals

- To alert the baby
- To calm the baby
- To engage the baby
- Increased vestibular stimulation to modify the baby's state
- Increased proprioceptive stimulation for postural control

10.2 Trunk-Pelvic-Hip Neutral Alignment: Weight Shifts

The goals of these facilitation techniques are to achieve trunk-pelvic-hip alignment in sitting, coactivate neck and trunk flexor muscles with neck and trunk extensor muscles, and facilitate sagittal plane righting reactions in the neck, trunk, and lower-extremity muscles.

You can use these techniques to examine the baby's ability to respond to anterior and posterior weight shifts. The response depends on the control of the appropriate muscles as well as the ability to receive and interpret the changes in the sensory feedback. If the baby does not respond, he or she will require further examination to determine if there is a motor control impairment or a sensory processing impairment.

It is important to consider which size ball will work best for the facilitation. If the baby is to remain on the ball, a very large one usually works best. If the baby will be transitioning off the ball, carefully consider the size according to the goal.

Baby's Position The baby sits on the ball facing you, with the hips in the center of the ball.

Therapist's Position Kneel in front of the baby, at or below eye level. You must be in a position that permits you to shift your weight with the baby and keep eye contact with the baby.

Therapist's Hands and Movement Place your hands on the baby's trunk and rest your arms on the ball and on the lateral aspects of the baby's femurs (figure 10.2.1). The contact of your arms on the baby's legs and the ball provides security to the baby and stability to the ball.

Align the baby's trunk and pelvis to a neutral and symmetrical position, and give downward pressure through the baby's trunk and pelvis into the ball.

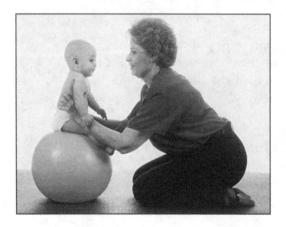

Figure 10.2.1. Trunk-pelvic-hip neutral alignment: Weight shifts. The therapist seats the baby on the ball facing her, with the baby's hips in the center of the ball. The therapist places her hands on the baby's trunk, resting her arms on the ball and on the lateral aspects of the baby's femurs, and aligns the baby's trunk and pelvis to a neutral and symmetrical position.

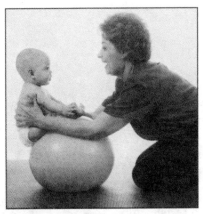

Figure 10.2.2. Posterior weight shift for activation of flexors. The therapist moves the baby and the ball backward while keeping the neutral alignment of the baby's trunk and pelvis and stabilizing the baby's trunk with her hands and the ball with her forearms. As the ball moves backward, the baby's trunk remains erect.

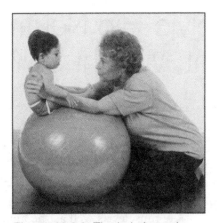

Figure 10.2.3. The baby's trunk flexes as the ball moves backward because the baby's trunk flexors activate without the trunk extensors. The therapist must correct this problem before going further with the facilitation technique.

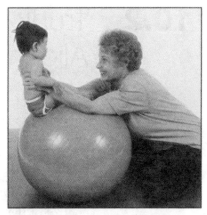

Figure 10.2.4. To correct trunk flexion, the therapist applies increased pressure with her fingers along the baby's spine to extend the spine.

Posterior Weight Shift for Activation of Flexors

Move the baby and the ball backward as you keep the neutral alignment of the baby's trunk and pelvis, and stabilize the baby's trunk with your hands and the ball with your forearms (figure 10.2.2).

As the ball moves backward, the baby's trunk must remain erect (figure 10.2.2). If the baby's trunk flexes (figure 10.2.3), correct this problem before going further with the facilitation technique. Apply increased pressure with your fingers along the baby's spine to extend the spine (figure 10.2.4).

When the ball moves backward, the baby should respond with a righting reaction to keep the trunk erect. To do this, the trunk flexors coactivate with the trunk extensors (figures 10.2.2 and 10.2.4). If the trunk flexors activate without the trunk extensors, the baby's trunk flexes (figure 10.2.3). The spine must remain erect so the movement occurs primarily at the hip joints.

Suggestion You may use downward pressure and subtle bouncing of the baby on the ball throughout the anterior-posterior movements to increase the baby's alertness or to calm the baby. Singing and eye contact are good ways to engage the baby.

Precautions

- Maintain your hand contact on the baby's trunk throughout the movements.
- Maintain your arm contact with the ball throughout the movements.

- Do not let the baby thrust backward.
- Do not let the baby collapse into flexion.

Component Goals
- Righting reactions into flexion with the hips, trunk, and head
- Balance of trunk extensors and flexors on the sagittal plane
- Rectus abdominus working off an extended spine
- Active chin tuck with elongation of the capital and cervical extensors
- Activation of the hip flexors
- Movement of the trunk and pelvis as a unit over the femurs

Functional Goals
- Activation of trunk muscles for sitting control
- Balance reactions during weight shifts in sitting

Anterior Weight Shift for Activation of Extensors

Keep the neutral alignment of the baby's trunk and pelvis, stabilize the baby's trunk with your hands and the ball with your fingers, and move the baby and the ball forward (figure 10.2.5).

As the ball moves forward, the baby's trunk must remain erect, and the hips must extend and stay on the ball (figure 10.2.5). When the ball moves forward, the baby should respond with righting reactions of head, trunk, and hip extension. The baby's trunk extensors must coactivate with the trunk flexors and hip extensors (figure 10.2.5). If the trunk extensors activate without the trunk flexors, the baby will fall backward. The spine must remain erect so that movement occurs primarily at the hip joints.

Babies who have difficulty with hip extension will try to lean forward at the hips when the ball rolls forward. If the baby tries to lean forward when the ball rolls forward, support the baby's trunk with your hands and **gently** apply backward pressure to the baby's chest with your thumbs (figure 10.2.6). Make sure you keep the baby's weight on the ball.

Forward to Symmetrical Stand

To bring the baby to stand, stabilize the baby's trunk and pelvis with your hands, and extend a few of your fingers to hold and stabilize the ball (figure 10.2.7). Stabilize the ball, the baby, and the baby on the ball, and roll the ball forward until the baby's feet reach the floor. When the baby's feet are on the ground, you can release the ball and move your fingers to the baby's hips to bring the baby to standing.

If the ball is too large for the baby's feet to reach the floor, continue the forward movement until the baby's feet rest on your legs, or continue the forward movement until the baby is "air standing." Air standing is

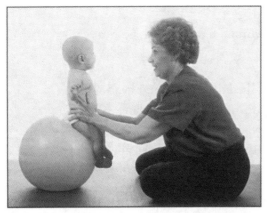

Figure 10.2.5. Anterior weight shift for activation of extensors. The therapist moves the baby and the ball forward, maintaining the neutral alignment of the baby's trunk and pelvis and stabilizing the baby's trunk with her hands and the ball with her forearms.

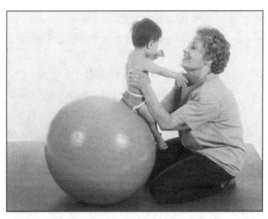

Figure 10.2.6. To keep the baby from leaning forward when the ball rolls forward, the therapist supports the baby's trunk with her hands and gently applies backward pressure to the baby's chest with her thumbs.

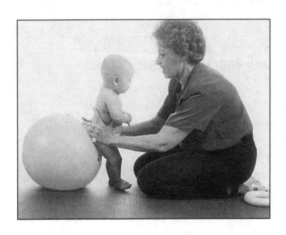

Figure 10.2.7. Forward to symmetrical stand. The therapist stabilizes the baby's trunk and pelvis with her hands, extending a few of her fingers to hold and stabilize the ball. The therapist then rolls the ball forward until the baby's feet reach the floor.

a position in which the baby is extended against the ball but the feet are not touching the floor (figures 10.2.5 and 10.2.6).

During the transition to stand, you must stabilize the baby's hips on the ball, and also stabilize the ball by keeping your fingers on the baby and the ball. Be careful that the ball does not push away as the baby's hips extend. If this is possible, place the ball near a wall or stabilize it with your feet.

Precautions

- Make sure you keep the baby's weight on the ball as it rolls forward.
- Stabilize the ball at all times with your arms, fingers, or feet.
- Do not permit the baby to use scapular adduction.
- Do not permit the baby to collapse and lean forward at the hips because of poor hip extensor control.

Component Goals

- Righting reactions into extension with the hips, trunk, and head
- Balance of trunk extensors and flexors on the sagittal plane
- Activation of the hip and knee extensors
- Downward protective extension reactions with the legs
- Movement of the trunk and pelvis as a unit over the femurs
- Lower-extremity weight bearing for standing

Functional Goals

- Preparation for standing
- Forward protective extension with the lower extremities
- Symmetrical standing

10.3 Lateral Weight Shifts for Simultaneous Activation of Flexors and Extensors

The goals of this technique are to facilitate lateral righting reactions, activate and balance the head and trunk flexors and extensors, and elongate the weight-bearing side. The trunk and hip muscles on the weight-bearing side work eccentrically while the trunk and hip muscles on the unweighted side work concentrically.

Therapists can use this technique to examine the baby's ability to respond to lateral movement of the center of mass. The response depends on control of the appropriate muscles, as well as the ability to receive and interpret the changes in the sensory feedback.

Baby's Position The baby sits on the ball, with the hips in the center of the ball. The feet do not touch the floor.

Therapist's Position Kneel in front of the baby, at or below eye level. You must be in an active position that permits you to shift your weight with the baby and keep eye contact with the baby.

Therapist's Hands Place your hands on the baby's trunk, and rest your arms on the ball or on the lateral aspects of the baby's femurs (figure 10.3.1). Your *guiding hand* is on the baby's weight-bearing side and your *assisting hand* is on the baby's unweighted side. The contact of your arms on the baby's legs and the ball provides security to the baby and stability to the ball. Your legs also may contact the ball to give you more control of the ball's movements.

Align the baby's trunk and pelvis to a neutral and symmetrical position and give downward pressure through the baby's trunk and pelvis into the ball to establish the base of support.

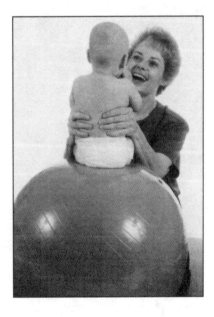

Figure 10.3.1. Lateral weight shifts for simultaneous activation of flexors and extensors. The therapist seats the baby on the ball facing her, with the baby's hips in the center of the ball. The therapist places her hands on the baby's trunk, resting her arms on the ball and on the lateral aspects of the baby's femurs.

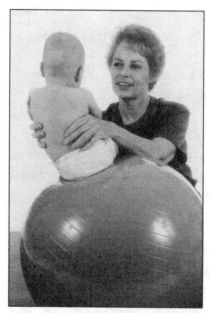 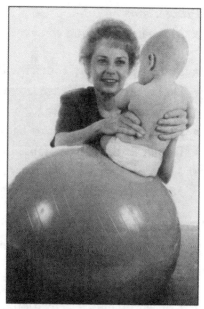

Figure 10.3.2. The therapist moves the baby and the ball sideward, stabilizing the baby's trunk with her hands and the ball with her arms. As the baby's weight moves laterally, the therapist uses her *guiding (right) hand* to help elongate the baby's weight-bearing side while her *assisting (left) hand* stabilizes and keeps the neutral alignment of the baby's trunk.

Figure 10.3.3. The therapist practices the weight shift to the opposite side. The therapist's *guiding (left) hand* elongates the baby's left side while her *assisting (right) hand* stabilizes and keeps the neutral alignment of the baby's trunk.

Movement Keep the neutral alignment of the baby's trunk and pelvis, stabilizing the baby's trunk with your hands and the ball with your arms, and move the baby and the ball sideward (figure 10.3.2).

When the ball moves sideward, the baby should respond with a lateral righting reaction to keep the trunk erect. The weight-bearing side elongates and the unweighted side laterally flexes. The trunk flexors and extensors on the weight-bearing side contract eccentrically, and the trunk flexors and extensors on the unweighted side contract concentrically.

As the baby's weight moves laterally, use your *guiding hand* to help elongate the baby's weight-bearing side (figures 10.3.2, 10.3.3).

Your *assisting hand* stabilizes and keeps the sagittal plane neutral alignment of the baby's trunk. **Do not** flex the baby's trunk laterally with your *assisting hand*. However, if the baby's trunk begins to rotate, apply **gentle** backward pressure with the thumb of your *assisting hand* to prevent trunk rotation.

Make sure you practice weight shifts to each side (figures 10.3.2, 10.3.3).

Precautions

- Maintain your hand contact on the baby's trunk throughout the movements.
- Maintain your arm contact with the ball throughout the movements.
- Do not shift the rib cage laterally over a stable pelvis.
- Do not rotate the rib cage.
- Do not let the baby thrust backward.
- Do not let the baby collapse into flexion.
- Make sure you keep the baby's weight on the ball as it rolls sideways.
- Maintain eye contact with the baby.

Component Goals

- Lateral righting of the trunk and head
- Balance of trunk extensors and flexors on the frontal plane
- Elongation with eccentric muscle activation of the weight-bearing side
- Concentric muscle activation on the unweighted side
- Pelvic-femoral (hip joint) mobility on the frontal plane

Functional Goals

- Lateral righting, used in upper-extremity sideward protective extension and reaching
- Lateral righting, used in movement transitions

10.4 Diagonal Weight Shifts: Rotation With Extension

The goals of these facilitation techniques are to increase the baby's ability to move on the transverse plane and to increase spinal mobility, pelvic-femoral mobility, upper-extremity protective extension, and upper-extremity weight bearing.

Baby's Position The baby sits on the peanut ball, with the hips in the center of the peanut ball. The feet do not touch the floor (figure 10.4.1). You also may use a ball for this technique.

Therapist's Position Sit in front of the baby with the peanut ball between your legs (figure 10.4.1). You must be in a position that permits you to shift your weight and have eye contact with the baby.

Therapist's Hands Place your hands laterally on the baby's trunk with the pads of your fingers near the baby's spine (figure 10.4.1). Rest your arms on the lateral aspects of the baby's legs to stabilize the baby and the peanut ball. If the baby has strong hip adduction, place your arms between the baby's legs.

Align the baby's trunk and pelvis to neutral on the sagittal plane and provide downward pressure through the baby's trunk and pelvis into the peanut ball.

Your *guiding hand* is on the baby's soon-to-be unweighted side. Your *assisting hand* is on the baby's soon-to-be weight-bearing side. (In figure 10.4.2, the therapist's right hand is the *guiding hand* and the left hand is the *assisting hand*.)

Movement While maintaining the neutral alignment of the trunk and pelvis, use your *guiding hand* to rotate one side of the baby's trunk and

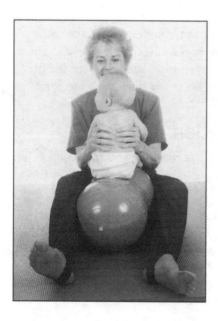

Figure 10.4.1. Diagonal weight shifts: Rotation with extension. The therapist sits in front of the baby on the peanut ball, seating the baby on the peanut ball with the hips in the center of the peanut ball. The therapist places her hands laterally on the baby's trunk, with the pads of her fingers near the baby's spine.

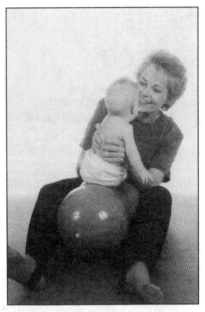

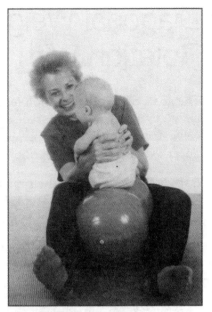

Figure 10.4.2. While maintaining the neutral alignment of the trunk and pelvis, the therapist uses her *guiding (right) hand* to rotate the left side of the baby's trunk and pelvis forward so that the baby's weight shifts to the right hip. The therapist's *assisting (left) hand* simultaneously rotates the right side of the trunk backward and maintains the alignment of the ribs over the pelvis.

Figure 10.4.3. Rotation in the opposite direction. While maintaining the neutral alignment of the trunk and pelvis, the therapist uses her *guiding (left) hand* to rotate the right side of the baby's trunk and pelvis forward so that the baby's weight shifts to the left hip. The therapist's *assisting (right) hand* simultaneously rotates the left side of the trunk backward and maintains the alignment of the ribs over the pelvis.

pelvis forward so that the baby's weight shifts to the opposite hip. (In figure 10.4.2, the baby's trunk rotates to the right and weight shifts to the right hip. In figure 10.4.3, the baby's trunk rotates to the left and weight shifts to the left hip.)

Your *assisting hand* simultaneously rotates the other side of the trunk backward and maintains the alignment of the ribs over the pelvis. The *assisting hand* prevents the rib cage from shifting laterally over the pelvis. The majority of the rotation movement occurs at the baby's hip joint.

Rotation With Hip Extension

When the baby feels comfortable with the rotation and the weight shift, you can reinforce the rotation by adding extension of the hip on the unweighted side (figure 10.4.4).

Once you have rotated the baby's trunk and pelvis, stabilize the baby's trunk with your *assisting hand* and move your *guiding hand* from the baby's trunk to the baby's unweighted leg (figure 10.4.4). Gently extend the baby's hip with your *guiding hand* as your *assisting hand* continues to rotate the baby's trunk. Internally rotate the baby's leg to increase

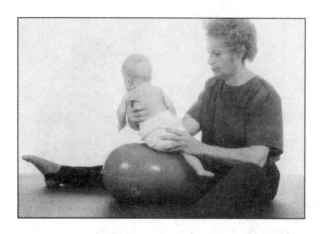

Figure 10.4.4. Rotation with hip extension. Having rotated the baby's trunk and pelvis, the therapist stabilizes the baby's trunk with her *assisting (right) hand* and moves her *guiding (left) hand* from the baby's trunk to the baby's unweighted leg. The therapist gently extends the baby's hip with her *guiding hand* as her *assisting hand* continues to rotate the baby's trunk. To increase the range into hip extension, the therapist internally rotates the baby's leg.

the range into hip extension. Most babies have limited range in hip extension and internal rotation. Therefore, do not force the baby to extend or rotate beyond what is comfortable. If the baby has full mobility for hip rotation, do not rotate the hip internally beyond neutral.

Modified Hand Placement If the baby has difficulty achieving and/or maintaining trunk extension, adduct the baby's arms to the trunk and stabilize them there (figure 10.4.5). Apply slight pressure with your thumbs to rotate the baby's humeri externally. External rotation of the humeri helps facilitate trunk extension (figure 10.4.5). Simultaneously apply inward pressure with the pads of your fingers along the baby's spine to extend the spine (figure 10.4.6).

When you have extended the baby's trunk, use both of your hands to maintain the adduction and external rotation of the baby's arms and rotate the baby to one side (figure 10.4.7). Your thumb provides a subtle backward pressure to the baby's shoulder girdle (figure 10.4.7). Shift your weight so that you maintain eye contact with the baby.

The baby's range of trunk rotation initially may appear to be more limited with the arms adducted to the side. However, the arm position enables the baby to achieve more thoracic spine extension and rotation rather than just lumbar spine mobility.

Upper-Extremity Weight Bearing

Baby's Position The baby sits on a ball, with the hips in the center of the ball. The feet do not touch the floor (figure 10.4.8).

Therapist's Position Heel-sit in front of the baby on the ball (figure 10.4.8). You must be in a position that permits you to shift your weight and have eye contact with the baby.

Therapist's Hands and Movement Use the modified hand placement to help the baby experience upper-extremity weight bearing. With your hands on the baby's arms, adduct them to the baby's sides with slight external rotation (figure 10.4.8). External rotation of the baby's arms

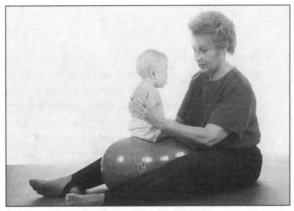

Figure 10.4.5. Modified hand placement. For the child with difficulty achieving and/or maintaining trunk extension, the therapist adducts the baby's arms to the trunk and stabilizes them there, applying slight pressure with her thumbs to rotate the baby's humeri externally.

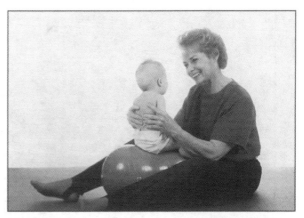

Figure 10.4.6. While adducting the baby's arms, the therapist simultaneously extends the baby's spine by applying inward pressure with the pads of her fingers along the baby's spine.

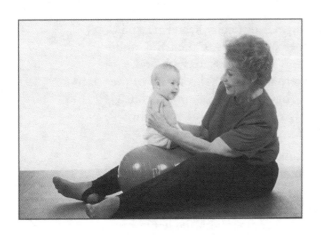

Figure 10.4.7. With the baby's trunk extended, the therapist uses both hands to maintain the adduction and external rotation of the baby's arms and rotates the baby to one side. The therapist's thumb provides a subtle backward pressure to the baby's shoulder girdle. The therapist shifts her weight to maintain eye contact with the baby.

helps facilitate trunk extension. Use the tips of your fingers on both hands to apply gentle pressure to extend the baby's trunk.

When you have extended the baby's trunk, use both of your hands to maintain adduction of the baby's arms and rotate the baby to one side (figure 10.4.9). As the baby rotates to the side, your *assisting (left) hand* places the baby's hand on the ball (figure 10.4.9). When the baby's hand is on the ball, use your *assisting hand* to externally rotate the baby's arm slightly. Your thumb provides a subtle backward pressure to the baby's shoulder girdle (figure 10.4.9).

Your *guiding (right) hand* stabilizes the baby on the ball and prevents the baby from retracting the unweighted arm (figure 10.4.10).

After the baby experiences upper-extremity weight bearing, you can maintain your hand placement and rotate the baby with a slightly faster speed to elicit upper-extremity protective extension. Make sure you continue to stabilize the baby throughout the movement.

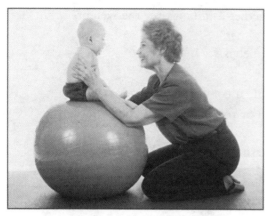

Figure 10.4.8. Upper-extremity weight bearing. The baby sits on the ball, and the therapist heel-sits in front of the baby. The therapist places her hands on the baby's arms and adducts them to the baby's sides with slight external rotation, using the tips of the fingers on both hands to apply gentle pressure to extend the baby's trunk.

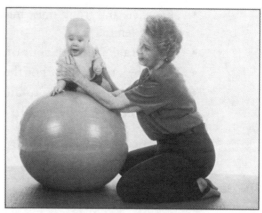

Figure 10.4.9. With the baby's trunk extended, the therapist uses both hands to maintain adduction of the baby's arms and rotates the baby to the right side. As the baby rotates to the right side, the therapist's *assisting (left) hand* places the baby's right hand on the ball and externally rotates the baby's arm slightly. The *assisting-hand thumb* provides a subtle backward pressure to the baby's shoulder girdle.

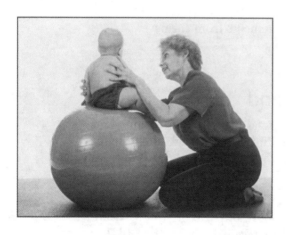

Figure 10.4.10. The therapist uses both hands to maintain adduction of the baby's arms and rotates the baby to the left side. The therapist's *guiding hand* stabilizes the baby on the ball and prevents the baby from retracting the unweighted arm.

Suggestions

- Your eye contact with the baby and your changing facial expressions can be very engaging for most babies.
- To involve the baby in the rotation, play a game where the baby looks for or at a toy on either side.
- The caregiver can stand behind the ball and move from side to side to motivate the baby to turn actively from side to side.
- Encourage the baby to initiate the head turning and rotation from side to side.

Precautions

- Maintain at least one hand on the baby's trunk at all times.
- Maintain one arm on the ball at all times.

- The pelvis and trunk must move together as a unit over the weight-bearing femur.
- The rib cage must not shift over the pelvis.
- The baby's trunk must not flex.
- Never force the baby to rotate beyond a comfortable range.
- Never force the baby's hip to extend or rotate beyond a comfortable range.
- Apply gentle pressure when you externally rotate the baby's humeri with your thumbs.

Component Goals

- Spinal extension with mobility on the transverse plane
- Activation of the trunk extensors
- Balance reactions with extension and rotation
- Upper-extremity weight bearing

Functional Goals

- Transverse plane mobility for exploration of the environment or retrieving toys when sitting
- Trunk mobility for transitions from sitting to quadruped or sitting to stand
- Balance control for transitional movements from sitting
- Upper-extremity protective extension

Rotation to One-Leg Stand

If the ball is small enough, you can extend the baby's unweighted leg and facilitate the baby to one-leg standing (figures 10.4.11 through 10.4.13). Change to a semilong-sitting position with the ball in front of you (figure 10.4.11).

Once the baby's weight shifts to the face-side leg and the unweighted leg extends (figure 10.4.11), use the elbow and arm of your *assisting hand* to stabilize the ball and the baby's face-side leg on the ball. It is important that your arm remain in contact with the ball in order to control the movement of the ball.

Use your *assisting hand* to stabilize the baby's trunk in the rotated position as you move your *guiding hand* from the baby's trunk to the baby's unweighted leg and extend the baby's hip (figure 10.4.12). Internally rotate the baby's hip to neutral to increase the range of hip extension. If the baby has difficulty with knee extension, place your *guiding hand* over the baby's knee and extend the baby's knee and hip.

Continue to stabilize the baby's trunk with your *assisting hand*, stabilize the ball with the arm of your *assisting hand*, and hold the baby's unweighted leg in extension with your *guiding hand*. Roll the ball laterally until the baby's foot is on the floor (figure 10.4.13).

When the baby's foot is on the floor, maintain the baby's hip and knee extension and press the baby's weight down to the heel of the foot with your *guiding hand*. The foot is the new base of support.

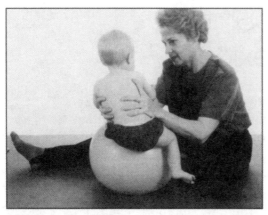

Figure 10.4.11. Rotation to one-leg stand. The therapist semilong-sits with the ball in front of her. With the baby's weight shifted to the face-side leg and the unweighted leg extended, the therapist uses the elbow and arm of her *assisting hand* to stabilize the ball and the baby's face-side leg on the ball.

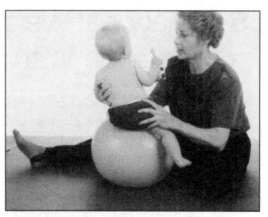

Figure 10.4.12. The therapist uses her *assisting (right) hand* to stabilize the baby's trunk in the rotated position as she moves her *guiding (left) hand* from the baby's trunk to the baby's unweighted leg and extends the baby's hip.

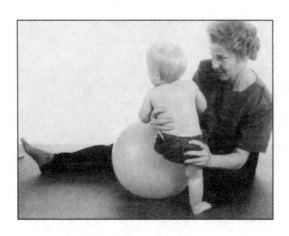

Figure 10.4.13. The therapist continues to stabilize the baby's trunk with her *assisting (right) hand*, stabilize the ball with the arm of her *assisting hand*, and hold the baby's unweighted leg in extension with her *guiding (left) hand* as she rolls the ball laterally until the baby's foot is on the floor.

Component Goals

- Spinal extension with mobility on the transverse plane
- Activation of the trunk extensors with the trunk flexors
- Lower-extremity dissociation
- Transverse plane mobility of the pelvis over the femur
- Pelvic-femoral (hip joint) mobility
- Hip extension with internal rotation to neutral
- Hip and knee extension for unilateral stance
- Lower-extremity weight bearing in single-limb stance

Functional Goals

- Single-limb stance in a midstance position
- Preparation for independent walking
- Dissociation of the lower extremities in preparation for stair climbing

10.5 Diagonal Weight Shifts: Rotation With Flexion

The goals of this facilitation are to activate and balance trunk flexors and extensors on a diagonal and facilitate balance reactions in sitting. The trunk and hip muscles work alternately between concentric and eccentric activity.

Therapists can use this technique to examine the baby's ability to respond to diagonal movement of the center of mass over the base of support. The response depends on control of the appropriate muscles, as well as the ability to receive and interpret the changes in the sensory feedback.

Baby's Position The baby sits on the ball, with the hips in the center of the ball. The feet do not touch the floor.

Therapist's Position Sit in front of the baby, at or below eye level, with the ball between your legs (figure 10.5.1). You also may kneel or stand in front of a very large ball. You must be in a position that permits you to shift your weight and have eye contact with the baby.

Therapist's Hands and Movement Place your hands laterally on the baby's rib cage and lower trunk (figure 10.5.1) and rest your arms on the ball. Align the baby's trunk and pelvis to neutral and apply downward pressure through the baby's trunk and pelvis into the ball.

Your *guiding hand* is on the baby's soon-to-be weight-bearing side. Your *assisting hand* is on the baby's soon-to-be unweighted side.

While maintaining the neutral alignment of the trunk and pelvis, move the baby diagonally backward on the ball, toward one hip (figure 10.5.2, baby's left hip). During the diagonal weight shift, use your *guiding hand* to elongate the baby's side by applying subtle traction to baby's trunk.

Use your *assisting hand* to shift the baby's weight diagonally backward to one hip and simultaneously rotate the baby's trunk backward on the unweighted side.

The diagonal weight shift should cause the baby to respond with trunk extension and elongation of the weight-bearing side, diagonal activation of the oblique abdominals, and rotation away from the weight shift. (In figure 10.5.2, the baby's weight shifts to the left and the baby rotates to the right. In figure 10.5.3, the baby's weight shifts to the right and the baby rotates to the left.)

Facilitate the diagonal weight shift to both sides (figures 10.5.2 and 10.5.3).

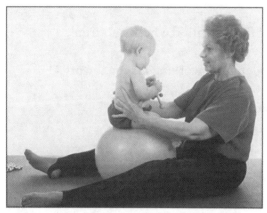

Figure 10.5.1. Diagonal weight shifts: Rotation with flexion. The baby sits on the ball with the hips in the center of the ball. The therapist places her hands laterally on the baby's rib cage and lower trunk and rests her arms on the ball, aligning the baby's trunk and pelvis to neutral and applying downward pressure through the baby's trunk and pelvis into the ball.

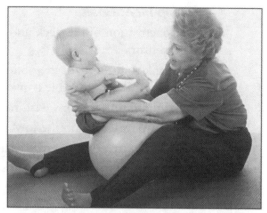

Figure 10.5.2. While maintaining the neutral alignment of the trunk and pelvis, the therapist moves the baby diagonally backward on the ball, toward the left hip, using her *guiding (right) hand* to elongate the baby's side by applying subtle traction to baby's trunk. The therapist's *assisting (left) hand* shifts the baby's weight diagonally backward to the left hip and simultaneously rotates the baby's trunk backward on the unweighted (right) side.

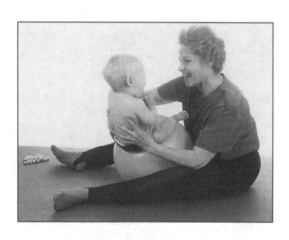

Figure 10.5.3. Rotation in the opposite direction: The baby's weight shifts to the right and the baby rotates to the left.

Precautions

- Move the ball diagonally backward. Do not move the ball sideward. Moving the ball sideward will cause the baby to flex laterally, lean, or sway into the ball.
- The pelvis and trunk must move together as a unit over the weight-bearing femur.
- The rib cage must not shift laterally over the pelvis.
- The rib cage must not rotate forward on the unweighted side.
- Although the weight shift activates the trunk flexors, the baby's trunk must extend, not flex.
- The pelvis must not rotate forward on the unweighted side.

Component Goals

- Coactivation of the neck and trunk flexors with the neck and trunk extensors
- Trunk rotation with the oblique abdominals working diagonally off an extended and stable trunk
- Equilibrium reactions with rotation in sitting
- Balance reactions in the lower extremities
- Upper-extremity forward reaching
- Activation of the pectoral muscles

Functional Goals

- Balance control for dressing activities
- Maintenance of balance when the center of mass is disturbed

11. Sitting on Bolster

11.1 Bench-Sitting on Bolster: Sagittal Plane Weight Shifts

The goals of these facilitation techniques are to achieve trunk-pelvic-hip alignment in sitting, coactivate neck and trunk flexor and extensor muscles, and facilitate sagittal plane righting reactions in the neck, trunk, and lower-extremity muscles.

Therapists can use these techniques to examine the baby's ability to respond to anterior and posterior weight shifts. The response depends on control of the appropriate muscles, as well as the ability to receive and interpret the changes in the sensory feedback. If the baby does not respond, the baby will require further evaluation to determine the presence of motor control or sensory processing impairments.

These techniques are similar to those described in Chapter 10, Sitting on Ball; however, the mobility of the bolster is more restricted. Therefore, the bolster may be preferable if you have difficulty controlling the baby or the ball.

Baby's Position   The baby bench-sits on the bolster facing you.

Therapist's Position   Kneel in front of the baby at, or below, eye level. You must be in a position that permits you to shift your weight with the baby.

Therapist's Hands and Movement   Place your hands on the baby's trunk, over the rib cage and pelvis, and rest your wrists or forearms on the baby's legs (figure 11.1.1). The contact of your arms on the baby's legs provides security to the baby.

Align the baby's trunk and pelvis to a neutral and symmetrical position to bring the shoulders directly into alignment over the hips, and give downward pressure through the baby's trunk and pelvis into the bolster.

Posterior Weight Shift for Activation of Flexors

While you maintain the neutral alignment of the baby's trunk and pelvis, stabilize the baby's trunk with your hands, and rest your forearms on the bolster next to the baby's legs. Move the baby and the bolster backward (figure 11.1.2).

As the bolster rolls backward, the baby's trunk must remain erect (figure 11.1.2). If the baby's trunk flexes, apply increased pressure with your fingers along the baby's spine to extend the spine.

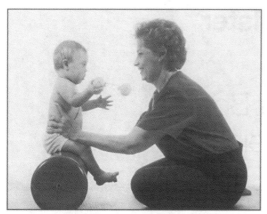

Figure 11.1.1. Bench-sitting on bolster: Sagittal plane weight shifts. The baby bench-sits on the bolster facing the therapist as she places her hands on the baby's trunk over the rib cage and pelvis, and rests her wrists on the baby's legs. The therapist aligns the baby's trunk and pelvis to a neutral and symmetrical position to bring the shoulders directly into alignment over the hips and gives downward pressure through the baby's trunk and pelvis into the bolster.

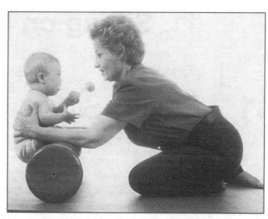

Figure 11.1.2. Posterior weight shift for activation of flexors. Maintaining the neutral alignment of the baby's trunk and pelvis, the therapist stabilizes the baby's trunk with her hands, and rests her forearms on the bolster next to the baby's legs as she moves the baby and the bolster backward.

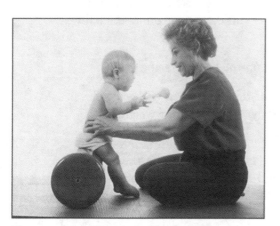

Figure 11.1.3. Anterior weight shift for activation of extensors. Maintaining the neutral alignment of the baby's trunk and pelvis, the therapist stabilizes the baby's trunk with her hands, and moves the baby and the bolster forward. The therapist supports the baby's trunk with her hands, and gently applies backward pressure to the baby's chest with her thumbs to keep the baby from leaning forward when the bolster rolls forward.

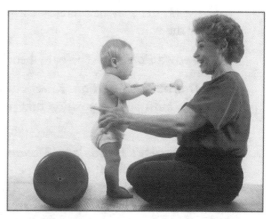

Figure 11.1.4. Forward to symmetrical stand. Once the baby's feet are on the floor, the therapist extends the baby's hips, and brings the baby to standing, continuing to stabilize the baby's trunk and hips.

When the bolster rolls backward, the baby should respond with a righting reaction to keep the trunk erect; the trunk flexors coactivate with the trunk extensors. If the trunk flexors activate without the trunk extensors, the baby's trunk will flex. The spine must remain erect so that the movement occurs primarily at the hip joints.

Anterior Weight Shift for Activation of Extensors

While you maintain the neutral alignment of the baby's trunk and pelvis, stabilize the baby's trunk with your hands and move the baby and the bolster forward (figure 11.1.3).

As the bolster rolls forward, the baby's trunk must remain erect, and the hips must extend and stay on the bolster (figure 11.1.3). When the bolster rolls forward, the baby should respond with a righting reaction to keep the trunk erect and extend the hips. To do this, the trunk extensors coactivate with the trunk flexors and hip extensors. If the trunk extensors activate without the trunk flexors, the baby will fall backward. The spine must remain erect so that the movement occurs primarily at the hip joints.

Babies who have difficulty with hip extension will try to lean forward at the hips when the bolster rolls forward. If this occurs, support the baby's trunk with your hands and **gently** apply backward pressure to the baby's chest with your thumbs (figure 11.1.3). Make sure you keep the baby's hips on the bolster.

Forward to Symmetrical Stand

To bring the baby to stand, stabilize the baby on the bolster, and roll it forward until the baby's feet reach the floor (figure 11.1.3). Once the baby's feet are on the floor, extend the baby's hips, and bring the baby to standing (figure 11.1.4). Continue to stabilize the baby's trunk and hips.

Suggestion Singing and eye contact are good ways to engage the baby.

Precautions

- Maintain your hand contact on the baby's trunk throughout the movements.
- Make sure you keep the baby's weight on the bolster as the bolster rolls.
- Do not let the baby thrust backward.
- Do not permit the baby to collapse and lean forward at the hips because of poor hip extensor control.

Component Goals

- Righting reactions into flexion and extension with the hips, trunk, and head
- Balance of trunk extensors and flexors on the sagittal plane
- Rectus abdominus working off an extended spine

- Activation of the hip flexors alternating with hip extensors
- Downward protective extension reactions with the legs
- Lower-extremity weight bearing for standing

Functional Goals
- Activation of trunk muscles for sitting control
- Balance reactions during weight shifts in sitting
- Trunk and hip muscle preparation for standing
- Forward protective extension with the lower extremities
- Symmetrical standing

11.2 Neutral Alignment of Trunk, Pelvis, and Hips

The goal of this technique is to facilitate neutral alignment of the baby's trunk, pelvis, and hips while sitting. Malalignment in one part of the body generates compensatory malalignment in other sections. Tightness in one joint leads to hypermobility in another joint.

Baby's Position The baby straddle-sits on a bolster, with the hips flexed to 90° and the knees flexed to 90° or less (figure 11.2.1). If the baby flexes the knees more than 90°, an anterior pelvic tilt will occur.

Therapist's Position Sit behind the baby.

Therapist's Hands and Movement If the baby is sitting with thoracic and lumbar flexion and a posterior pelvic tilt (figure 11.2.1), place both hands on the baby's trunk with your thumbs near the baby's spine. Gently press in with your thumbs and extend the baby's spine as you extend the baby's rib cage with your hands (figure 11.2.2). Once you have extended the baby's trunk, apply subtle downward pressure through the rib cage into the pelvis. Be careful not to flex the baby's trunk when you press down.

To increase the baby's trunk extension, stabilize the baby's trunk with your *guiding hand* and move your *assisting hand* to the baby's arm

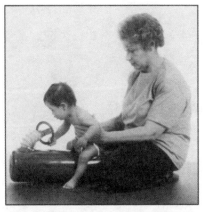

Figure 11.2.1. Neutral alignment of trunk, pelvis, and hips. The baby straddle-sits on a bolster with the hips flexed to 90° and the knees flexed to 90° or less. To correct thoracic and lumbar flexion and a posterior pelvic tilt, the therapist places both hands on the baby's trunk with her thumbs near the baby's spine.

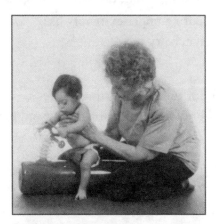

Figure 11.2.2. The therapist gently presses in with her thumbs and extends the baby's spine as she extends the baby's rib cage with her hands, applying subtle downward pressure through the rib cage into the pelvis once she has extended the baby's trunk.

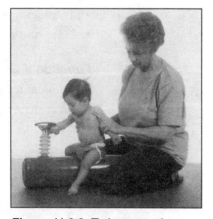

Figure 11.2.3. To increase the baby's trunk extension, the therapist stabilizes the baby's trunk with her *guiding (right) hand*, using the thumb of her *guiding hand* to continue to apply gentle pressure near the baby's spine as her fingers stabilize the rib cage in extension. The therapist grasps the baby's arm with her *assisting (left) hand*, adducting, externally rotating, and applying slight backward pressure to the baby's humerus.

(figure 11.2.3). The thumb of your *guiding hand* continues to apply gentle pressure near the baby's spine as your fingers stabilize the rib cage in extension.

Grasp the baby's arm with your *assisting hand;* adduct, externally rotate, and apply a slight backward pressure to the baby's humerus (figure 11.2.3). Humeral external rotation helps facilitate trunk extension.

Once the baby's trunk and pelvis are in neutral alignment, you can facilitate movements in different directions.

Suggestions

- This is a good technique to use for helping the baby maintain trunk extension while using one hand (figure 11.2.3).
- Use suction toys that stick on the bolster to engage the baby in active play.

Precautions

- Do not elevate the baby's rib cage when you extend the trunk.
- Make sure the pressure with your thumb is gentle.
- Externally rotate the baby's arm only as far as is comfortable for the baby.

Component Goals

- Thoracic extension mobility to neutral from flexion
- Neutral alignment of the spine and head on the pelvis
- Neutral alignment of the pelvis over the femurs
- Trunk extension during upper-extremity use
- Head and trunk symmetry

Functional Goals

- Trunk extension for functional sitting
- Erect sitting posture for all upper-extremity and oral-motor activities

11.3 Sitting on Bolster: Anterior Weight Shifts

Many babies with movement problems do not move from the hip joints when reaching forward and when rising to stand. They often compensate and move forward from the thoracic spine and increase their kyphosis, or they move from the lumbar spine and increase their anterior pelvic tilt and lordosis.

The goal of this facilitation technique is to increase the baby's ability to move from the hip joints when reaching forward and when rising to stand. Additional goals include pelvic-femoral mobility on the sagittal plane, active spinal extension, and synchronous movement of the baby's trunk and pelvis forward over the femurs.

Baby's Position The baby straddle-sits on a bolster, with the hips flexed to 90° and the knees flexed to 90° or less (figure 11.3.1). Flexion of the baby's knees to more than 90° will produce an anterior pelvic tilt.

The spine is neutral (or as close to neutral as possible) on the sagittal plane. (See the previous facilitation, 11.2, Neutral Alignment of Trunk, Pelvis, and Hips.) Flexion or extension of the spine in one section will cause hypermobility at another point. This is frequently a problem in babies with movement disorders.

Place the bolster in a flat or inclined position.

Therapist's Position Sit behind the baby.

Therapist's Hands and Movement Depending on the baby's needs, you can facilitate forward weight shifts from various control points. You can enhance the forward movement of the baby's trunk by having the baby reach forward with shoulder flexion for an object or activity at or above shoulder level. If you incline the bolster, you can place toys at the top of the bolster.

Facilitation From the Trunk

If the baby has independent use of the arms and can reach up for the toys but has difficulty moving the trunk and pelvis as a unit (as is the case with many babies who have low tone), use your hands to align and stabilize the baby's rib cage and pelvis together. Place your hands on the baby's trunk and spread your fingers between the baby's rib cage and pelvis (figure 11.3.2).

If the baby has lumbar hyperextension, apply subtle pressure to the baby's rib cage with your index and middle fingers, then bring the rib cage posterior and align it with the pelvis. This will flex the lumbar spine to neutral. Do not flex the spine beyond neutral, because this will cause a posterior pelvic tilt and a kyphosis.

If the baby has lumbar flexion, apply subtle pressure to the baby's posterior rib cage with your thumbs, then bring the rib cage forward

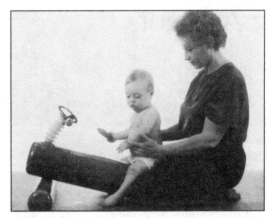

Figure 11.3.1. Sitting on bolster: Anterior weight shifts. The baby straddle-sits on a bolster with the hips flexed to 90° and the knees flexed to 90° or less.

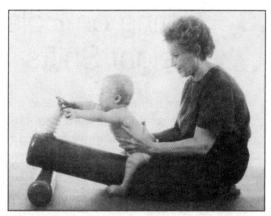

Figure 11.3.2. Facilitation from the trunk. The therapist stabilizes the baby's rib cage and pelvis together, placing her hands on the baby's trunk and spreading her fingers between the baby's rib cage and pelvis. The therapist then moves the baby's trunk forward at the hip joints as the baby reaches forward with both arms.

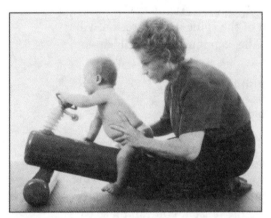

Figure 11.3.3. Facilitation from the trunk: Rise to stand. With the baby's feet on the floor, the therapist keeps her fingers on the baby's anterior trunk and maintains the alignment of the rib cage to the pelvis as the baby reaches forward. The therapist moves her thumbs to the baby's hips, using her thumbs to help the baby shift the weight forward onto the legs.

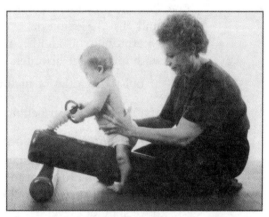

Figure 11.3.4. When the baby's weight is on the legs and the gluteus maximus actively contracts, the therapist continues to use her fingers to facilitate the baby's trunk toward the upright posture.

and align it with the pelvis. This will extend the lumbar spine to neutral. Do not extend the spine beyond neutral; this causes an anterior pelvic tilt.

While maintaining neutral alignment of the rib cage and pelvis, move the baby's trunk forward at the hip joints as the baby reaches forward with both arms (figure 11.3.2). Maintain the baby's trunk alignment during the forward reach and when the baby returns to neutral sitting. Make sure that the baby moves at the hip joints.

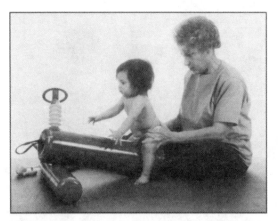

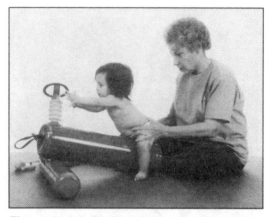

Figure 11.3.5. Facilitation from the pelvis. The therapist places her hands on the lateral aspects of the baby's pelvis, thumbs on the posterior aspects of the pelvis. The therapist stabilizes the baby's femurs with her fourth and fifth fingers.

Figure 11.3.6. As the baby reaches forward with the arms, the therapist uses her thumbs to guide the baby's pelvis forward over the femurs, being careful to keep the pelvis and trunk aligned.

Rise to Stand

To facilitate the baby's rising to stand, place the baby's feet on the floor (figure 11.3.2). As the baby reaches forward, keep your fingers on the baby's anterior trunk and maintain the alignment of the rib cage to the pelvis. Move your thumbs to the baby's hips, and use your thumbs to help the baby shift the weight forward onto the legs (figure 11.3.3).

When the baby's weight is on the legs, continue to facilitate the baby's hip extension with your thumbs while you use your fingers to facilitate the baby's trunk toward the upright posture (figure 11.3.4). Continue the pressure with your thumbs and fingers until the baby rises to standing and the gluteus maximus actively contracts. When the baby is standing, maintain the pressure on the baby's rib cage and hips. You may move your thumb from the baby's hips to the baby's trunk if the baby actively contracts the gluteus maximus (figure 11.3.4).

Facilitation From the Pelvis

If the baby has some independent use of the arms and some upper trunk control but has difficulty moving the pelvis over the femurs, place your hands on the lateral aspects of the baby's pelvis, with your thumbs on the posterior aspects of the pelvis (figure 11.3.5).

As the baby reaches forward with the arms, use your thumbs to guide the baby's pelvis forward over the femurs (figure 11.3.6). You can stabilize the baby's femurs with your fourth and fifth fingers (figures 11.3.5 and 11.3.6). Stabilization of the femurs is especially important if the baby's legs tend to abduct and/or extend.

Be careful: forward movement of the pelvis must not go so far as to cause an anterior pelvic tilt with lumbar extension. The pelvis and trunk must remain aligned (figure 11.3.6).

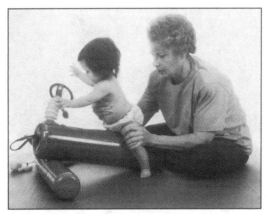

Figure 11.3.7. Facilitation from the pelvis: Rise to stand. As the baby reaches forward, the therapist moves her hands from the baby's pelvis to the baby's femurs, placing her fingers on the femurs and thumbs on the baby's hips. The therapist presses up and in with her thumbs to extend the baby's hips while her fingers stabilize the baby's femurs and press weight down into the baby's feet. The therapist has moved one hand from the baby's femur to the baby's anterior rib cage and aligned the rib cage and the pelvis, to prevent anterior pelvic tilt and hyperextension of the lumbar spine and to shift the baby's weight backward until the trunk is over the pelvis and legs.

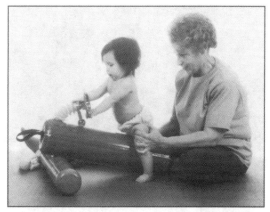

Figure 11.3.8. When the baby can maintain this posture, the therapist returns her hand to the baby's femur so that both of her hands are on the baby's femurs and her thumbs are on the baby's hips. The therapist then applies upward and inward pressure with her thumbs to extend the baby's hips and applies downward pressure with her hands while her fingers externally rotate the baby's femurs to transfer weight to the lateral borders of the feet.

Rise to Stand

To facilitate the baby's rising to stand, place the baby's feet on the floor (figure 11.3.6). As the baby reaches forward, move your hands from the baby's pelvis to the baby's femurs (figure 11.3.7). Place your fingers on the femurs and your thumbs on the baby's hips. Press up and in with your thumbs to extend the baby's hips while your fingers stabilize the baby's femurs and press weight down into the baby's feet.

If the baby's lumbar spine hyperextends, or an anterior pelvic tilt occurs, move one hand from the baby's femur to the baby's anterior rib cage and align the rib cage and the pelvis (figure 11.3.7). Keep your other hand on the baby's femur with your thumb on the baby's hip.

Use your hand on the baby's trunk to shift the baby's weight backward until the trunk is over the pelvis and legs. When the baby can maintain this posture, return your hand to the baby's femur so that both of your hands are on the baby's femurs and your thumbs are on the baby's hips (figure 11.3.8).

When both of your hands are on the baby's femurs, apply upward and inward pressure with your thumbs to extend the baby's hips. Apply downward pressure with your hands while your fingers externally rotate the baby's femurs to transfer weight to the lateral borders of the feet (figure 11.3.8).

Precautions

- The trunk and pelvis must remain in a neutral position on the sagittal plane when moving forward.
- The rib cage and pelvis must move as a unit.
- The movement must occur at the hip joints, that is, pelvis over femurs.
- Do not enable the thoracic spine to flex during the movement.
- Do not enable the lumbar spine to flex or hyperextend.
- Do not enable the pelvis to tilt anteriorly or posteriorly.

Component Goals

- Shoulder flexion with upper-extremity reaching
- Trunk extension
- Forward movement of the trunk and pelvis over the femurs
- Pelvic-femoral (hip joint) mobility on the sagittal plane
- Graded control of the quadriceps for knee extension
- Elongation of the hamstring and gastrocnemius muscles when standing
- Eccentric activity of the hip extensors

Functional Goals

- Increased hip and trunk control for forward reaching in sitting
- Increased pelvic-femoral (hip joint) mobility and control for forward transitions, such as coming to stand from sitting, or floor sitting to quadruped

Lateral Weight Shifts in Standing

Once the baby is stable in standing, you can practice lateral weight shifts to single-limb stance to prepare the baby for walking.

Place your hands on the lateral sides of the baby's hip joints so that your fingers are on the baby's femurs and your thumbs are on the gluteus maximus (figure 11.3.8). Do not place your fingers on the baby's hip flexors.

Your *guiding hand* is on the hip of the baby's soon-to-be weight-bearing leg (figure 11.3.9, therapist's left hand). Your *assisting hand* is on the opposite hip (figure 11.3.9, therapist's right hand).

Use both of your hands to shift the baby's weight laterally onto one leg. As the baby's weight shifts, use the thumb of your *guiding hand* to apply subtle upward pressure on the baby's gluteus maximus to facilitate hip extension while the fingers of your *guiding hand* stabilize the baby's femur and press weight down into the baby's foot (figure 11.3.9).

Use your *assisting hand* to shift the baby's weight laterally, flex the baby's unweighted hip and knee, and lift the baby's leg until the baby's foot rests on the bolster (figures 11.3.9 and 11.3.10).

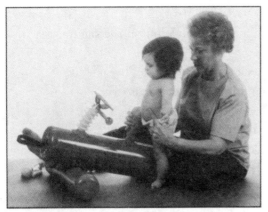

Figure 11.3.9. Lateral weight shifts in standing. The therapist uses both hands to shift the baby's weight laterally onto one leg. As the baby's weight shifts, the therapist uses her *guiding (left) hand* to stabilize the baby's hip and leg in the extended and weight-bearing position, applying subtle upward pressure with her thumb on the baby's gluteus maximus to facilitate hip extension. The therapist uses her *assisting (right) hand* to shift the baby's weight laterally, flex the baby's unweighted hip and knee, and lift the baby's leg until the baby's foot rests on the bolster.

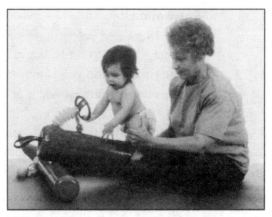

Figure 11.3.10. The therapist practices the lateral weight shift to the opposite side.

Make sure that you practice the lateral weight shifts to both sides (figures 11.3.9 and 11.3.10).

Precautions

- The trunk and pelvis must remain in a neutral position on the sagittal plane when moving laterally.
- The rib cage and pelvis must move as a unit over the hip.
- The movement must occur at the hip joint.
- Do not enable the thoracic spine to flex laterally during the movement.

Component Goals

- Trunk extension
- Graded control of the quadriceps for knee extension
- Eccentric activity of the hip abductors and extensors

Functional Goals

- Lateral weight shifts for walking
- Balance control in standing

11.4 Half-Kneeling From a Bolster

The goals of these facilitation techniques are to increase the baby's trunk, hip, and lower-extremity mobility and control for half-kneeling and to increase the baby's balance in half-kneeling. The ultimate functional goal is for the baby to move independently from the floor to standing by transitioning from kneeling to half-kneeling to standing.

Baby's Position   The baby sits straddling a bolster, with hips and knees at 90° (figure 11.4.1). The baby's knees should not flex more than 90°.

The bolster must be the same height as the baby's femur. If the bolster is too big, the baby will not be able to half-kneel around the bolster. A bolster that is too small will not provide the needed support for lower-extremity dissociation.

Therapist's Position   Sit behind the baby.

Therapist's Hands and Movement   The transition to half-kneeling begins with trunk/spinal rotation with extension. The bolster facilitates lower-extremity dissociation.

Place both of your hands on the baby's rib cage and align the trunk on the sagittal plane (figure 11.4.1). Your hand on the baby's anterior rib cage is the *assisting hand;* your hand on the baby's back is the *guiding hand.* If the baby's trunk is flexed, use both of your hands to extend the baby's trunk. Maintain the baby's trunk extension, and give downward pressure into the pelvis and hips to reinforce awareness of the base of support.

When you have extended the baby's trunk and aligned the rib cage and pelvis, use your *guiding hand* to rotate the baby's trunk (figure 11.4.2). Rotation of the spine must facilitate rotation of the pelvis over the face-side femur. Do not simply rotate the rib cage over a stable pelvis. This will create mobility and possibly hypermobility in the spine.

If the baby tries to retract the shoulder as the trunk rotates forward, use the fingers of your *guiding hand* to hold the baby's arm forward (figure 11.4.2).

Use your *assisting hand* to assist the baby's trunk to rotate and to keep the baby's rib cage aligned with the pelvis. Do not let the baby's rib cage rotate without the pelvis, and do not let it shift laterally over the pelvis. Do not pull the baby's rib cage backward with your *assisting hand.*

Once the baby's trunk has rotated, and the weight has shifted to the face-side leg, move your *assisting hand* to the baby's far arm and hold it forward (figure 11.4.3). Move your *guiding hand* to the baby's unweighted leg, grasping the tibia near the knee with your fingers and aligning your thumb vertically on the femur (figure 11.4.3). Use your *guiding hand* to extend and rotate the baby's hip internally to neutral while flexing the knee and placing it on the floor (figure 11.4.4). Weight bearing on the bolster will maintain the baby's forward leg in flexion.

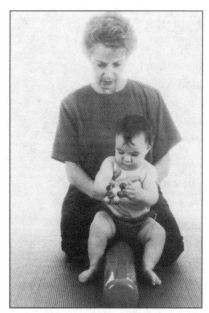

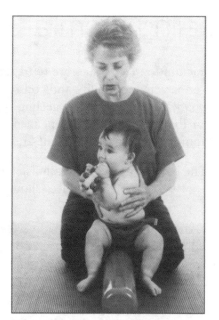

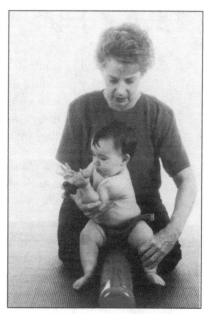

Figure 11.4.1. Half-kneeling from a bolster. The baby straddle-sits on a bolster with the hips flexed to 90° and the knees flexed to 90° or less. The therapist places her *guiding hand* on the baby's back and her *assisting hand* on the baby's anterior rib cage, using both hands to align the trunk on the sagittal plane.

Figure 11.4.2. The therapist uses her *guiding (left) hand* to rotate the baby's trunk. The fingers of the therapist's *guiding hand* hold the baby's arm forward to prevent shoulder retraction as the trunk rotates forward. The therapist's *assisting (right) hand* assists the baby's trunk to rotate and keeps the baby's rib cage aligned with the pelvis.

Figure 11.4.3. With the baby's trunk rotated and the weight shifted to the face-side leg, the therapist moves her *assisting (right) hand* to the baby's far arm to hold it forward and moves her *guiding (left) hand* to the baby's back leg, grasping the tibia near the knee with her fingers and aligning her thumb vertically on the femur.

Once the baby's knee is on the floor in a weight-bearing position, move your *guiding hand* to the baby's hip to stabilize the hip (figure 11.4.5). Use your *assisting hand* on the baby's arm or anterior rib cage to shift the baby's trunk over the weight-bearing hip (figure 11.4.5). If the baby keeps both arms forward, move your *assisting hand* to the baby's anterior rib cage to stabilize the trunk in an extended position.

Posterior Weight Shifts
Support the baby in half-kneeling with your *assisting hand* on the baby's anterior rib cage and your *guiding hand* on the baby's extended hip (see figure 11.4.5). While maintaining this position, guide the baby's weight backward with your *assisting hand* (figure 11.4.6). Use your *guiding hand* to keep the pelvis and weight-bearing femur aligned as the baby's weight moves backward (figure 11.4.6).

As the baby's weight moves backward, the bolster elongates the hamstrings of the baby's forward leg (figure 11.4.6).

Anterior Weight Shifts
Support the baby in half-kneeling with your *assisting hand* on the baby's anterior rib cage and your *guiding hand* on the baby's extended hip (see figure 11.4.5).

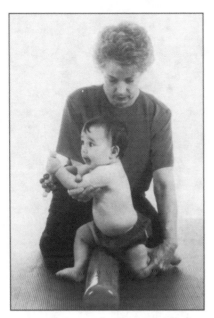 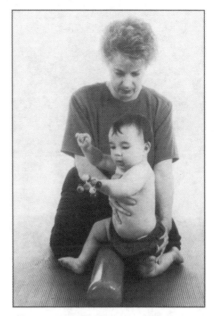

Figure 11.4.4. The therapist uses her *guiding hand* to extend and rotate the baby's hip internally to neutral while flexing the knee and placing it on the floor.

Figure 11.4.5. With the baby's knee on the floor in a weight-bearing position, the therapist moves her *guiding (left) hand* to the baby's hip to stabilize the hip, using her *assisting (right) hand* on the baby's arm and anterior rib cage to shift the baby's trunk over the weight-bearing hip.

While maintaining this position, slide your *guiding hand* from the baby's hip to the baby's femur and extend the baby's hip and knee as you guide the baby's weight forward with your *assisting hand* (figure 11.4.7). The baby can reach forward and up or forward and down to retrieve a toy.

Make sure you stabilize the baby's hip and knee in extension before the weight shifts forward, otherwise the baby will pull the leg into flexion very quickly.

Return to Sitting
Return the baby to sitting on the bolster by using your *assisting hand* to rotate the trunk back to its original erect position.

Component Goals
- Trunk and pelvic rotation over the femur
- Lower-extremity dissociation
- Pelvic-femoral (hip joint) mobility on all three planes
- Activation of all hip muscles
- Hip extension, internal rotation to neutral, and adduction to neutral on the back leg
- Elongation of hip flexors and knee extensors on the back leg
- Hip flexion, external rotation to neutral, and adduction to neutral on the front leg

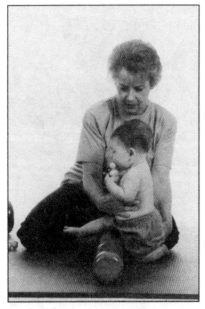

Figure 11.4.6. Posterior weight shifts. Supporting the baby in half-kneeling, the therapist guides the baby backward with her *assisting (right) hand* and stabilizes the weight-bearing hip with her *guiding (left) hand*.

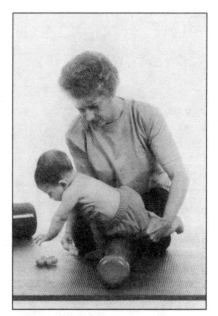

Figure 11.4.7. Anterior weight shifts. Supporting the baby in half-kneeling, the therapist slides her *guiding (left) hand* from the baby's hip to the baby's femur and extends the baby's hip and knee as she guides the baby's weight forward with her *assisting (right) hand*.

- Elongation of hip and knee extensors on the front leg
- Elongation of the hip adductors on both legs
- Elongation of the hamstrings on the forward leg during posterior weight shifts
- Elongation of the hip flexors on the back leg during forward weight shifts
- Forward movement of the tibia over the forward foot

Functional Goals

- Lower-extremity mobility, in preparation for the transition from kneeling to half-kneeling
- Movement of the trunk and pelvis over the lower extremities in preparation for use in higher-level transitions
- Rising to stand from half-kneeling with graded knee extension

11.5 Rotation to Step Stance: Face-Side Weight Shift

The goals of these facilitation techniques are to prepare the baby's trunk, pelvis, and lower extremities for the transition from sitting to standing and to prepare for transitions in stepping.

Baby's Position The baby sits straddling a bolster, with hips and knees at 90° (figure 11.5.1). The baby's knees should not flex more than 90°.

Therapist's Position Sit behind the baby.

Therapist's Hands and Movement Use both of your hands to stabilize the baby and align the baby's trunk, legs, and arms on the bolster (figure 11.5.1).

When the baby is stable, place the arm of your *assisting hand* under the baby's near arm and grasp the baby's far arm with your *assisting hand* (figure 11.5.2). Support the baby's trunk with the arm of your *assisting hand*. Use your *assisting hand and arm* to rotate the baby's trunk and shift the baby's weight to the face side (figure 11.5.2). Be careful to rotate the pelvis with the rib cage.

Place your *guiding hand* on the baby's rib cage and use it to maintain the alignment of the rib cage and pelvis during the rotation (figure 11.5.2).

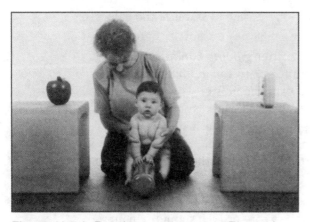

Figure 11.5.1. Rotation to step stance: Face-side weight shift. The baby straddle-sits on a bolster. The therapist uses both of her hands to stabilize the baby and align the baby's trunk, legs, and arms on the bolster with the hips flexed to 90° and the knees flexed to 90° or less.

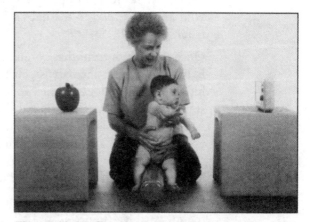

Figure 11.5.2. The therapist rotates the baby's trunk and shifts the baby's weight to the face side. She places the arm of her *assisting (left) hand* under the baby's near arm and grasps the baby's far arm with her *assisting hand* while supporting the baby's trunk with the arm of her *assisting hand*. She uses her *assisting hand* and arm to rotate the baby's trunk, being careful to rotate the pelvis with the rib cage. The therapist uses her *guiding (right) hand* to maintain the alignment of the baby's rib cage and pelvis during the rotation.

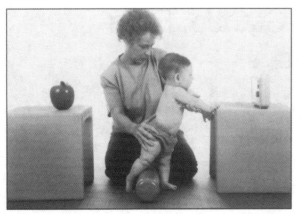

Figure 11.5.3. Single-limb stance: Forward leg. The therapist uses her *assisting (left) hand* to guide the baby to rise to single-limb standing while maintaining the baby's trunk rotation and extension. The therapist slides her *guiding (right) hand* to the baby's pelvis and femur to ensure that the baby's hip extends and does not flex forward over the bolster.

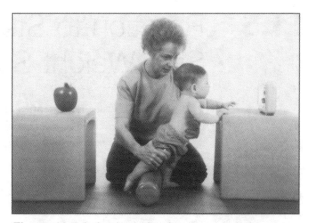

Figure 11.5.4. As the baby rises to stand, the therapist slides her *guiding (right) hand* down the baby's back leg, grasping the femur near the knee with her fingers and aligning her thumb vertically on the femur. The *guiding hand* extends and internally rotates the baby's hip to neutral while extending the knee; it also shifts and keeps the baby's weight forward on the forward leg. The therapist moves her *assisting (left) hand* to the baby's anterior rib cage to stabilize the baby's trunk.

Single-Limb Stance: Forward Leg

Once the baby's trunk rotates, and the weight shifts to the face-side leg, encourage the baby to reach up for a toy with both hands. Use your *assisting hand* to guide the baby to rise to single-limb standing while maintaining the baby's trunk rotation and extension (figure 11.5.3). As the baby rises to stand, place the baby's hands on the bench and move your *assisting hand* to the baby's anterior rib cage to stabilize the baby's trunk (figure 11.5.4).

Once the baby's trunk has rotated, slide your *guiding hand* from the baby's rib cage to the baby's pelvis and femur to ensure that the baby's hip extends and does not flex forward over the bolster when rising to stand (figure 11.5.3). As the baby rises to stand, slide your *guiding hand* down the baby's back leg, grasping the femur near the knee with your fingers and aligning your thumb vertically on the femur (figure 11.5.4). Use your *guiding hand* to extend and rotate the baby's hip internally to neutral while extending the knee (figure 11.5.4).

Use your *guiding hand* to shift and keep the baby's weight forward on the forward leg (figure 11.5.4). The baby's forward leg should remain extended at the hip and knee. Repeat this movement several times, rotating from side to side.

Suggestion Having the baby reach up for a toy on a stable surface will assist the weight shift.

Precautions Do not rotate the baby's trunk by just pulling on the baby's arms.

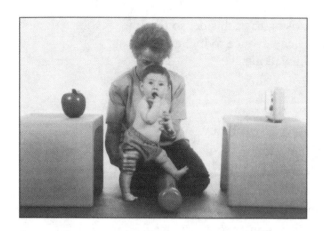

Figure 11.5.5. Single-limb stance: Back leg. The therapist uses her *assisting (left) hand* to guide the baby's trunk backward over the leg. At the same time, she uses her *guiding (right) hand* to keep the hip and knee extended while pressing the leg down and back until the baby's heel is on the floor. Once the foot is in a weight-bearing position, the therapist's *guiding hand* externally rotates the baby's femur to shift the baby's weight to the lateral border of the foot. The thumb of the therapist's *guiding hand* presses toward the baby's hip to maintain the hip extension.

Component Goals

- Pelvic-femoral (hip joint) mobility, especially rotation
- Elongation of the hip adductors on both legs
- Graded control of the quadriceps (forward leg)
- Weight bearing on the foot in neutral alignment (forward leg)
- Trunk extension
- Forward progression of the pelvis and trunk over the forward leg

Functional Goals

- Rising to stand from sitting
- Forward weight shift to one-leg stance
- Foot and lower-extremity preparation for midstance transitions

Single-Limb Stance: Back Leg

From the forward position, you can shift the baby's weight posteriorly to the back foot (figures 11.5.4 and 11.5.5).

To shift the baby's weight to the back leg, maintain the baby's hip and knee in extension with neutral hip rotation, apply slight backward traction, and place the toes of the baby's back foot on the floor with your *guiding hand*. Continue to extend and support the baby's trunk and arms with your *assisting hand*. (See figure 11.5.4 for placement of the therapist's hands and the baby's foot.)

Once the baby's toes are on the floor, use your *assisting hand* to guide the baby's trunk backward over the leg. At the same time, use your *guiding hand* to keep the hip and knee extended while you press the leg down and back until the baby's heel is on the floor (figure 11.5.5).

When the baby's foot is in a flat, weight-bearing position and the trunk is aligned and erect over the foot, use your *guiding hand* to rotate the baby's femur externally, so that the baby's weight shifts to the lateral border of the foot. Press the thumb of your *guiding hand* toward the baby's hip to maintain the hip extension.

As the baby's weight shifts backward, the forward leg unweights and rests on the bolster. The baby's hamstring muscles elongate as the knee extends while supported by the bolster (figure 11.5.5).

Practice this technique by rotating and rising to each side, so that the baby's mobility and control increase. Then advance to higher-level gait techniques to increase the baby's skill in walking.

Component Goals

- Trunk extension
- Pelvic-femoral (hip joint) mobility, especially rotation
- Elongation of the hip adductors on both legs
- Elongation of the hamstrings on the front leg during the posterior weight shift
- Elongation of the gastrocnemius and toe flexors
- Hip and knee extension on the back leg, similar to midstance
- Weight bearing on the foot in neutral alignment (back leg)

Functional Goals

- Foot and lower-extremity preparation for midstance transitions
- Foot and lower-extremity preparation for terminal stance, pre-swing (back leg)
- Swing position of the forward leg (posterior weight shift)

12. Standing and Walking

When babies begin to pull to stand, they typically practice movements on the sagittal, frontal, and transverse planes while standing. These movements help prepare the baby for independent walking.

The baby typically begins to practice **sagittal plane** movements in standing by bouncing up and down, that is, hip and knee flexion without the feet leaving the ground. Once the baby can pull to stand independently, the baby practices sagittal plane movements by transitioning from standing to sitting or squatting. The baby begins with a very limited range of hip and knee flexion and progresses to full flexion. These sagittal plane movements rely on and help develop eccentric-concentric muscle control in the lower extremities, especially the quadriceps and hip extensors.

The baby practices **frontal plane** movements in standing by shifting weight to one leg, then the other. Lateral weight shifts help the baby develop hip abductor, adductor, and extensor control. Lateral weight shifts also help the baby develop inversion and eversion control in the foot. The baby spends a lot of time practicing frontal plane control by cruising around the furniture.

The baby practices **transverse plane** movements in standing by rotating the trunk and pelvis. When lateral rotation of the trunk and pelvis occurs on a weight-bearing leg, the femur and tibia externally rotate. This subsequently results in transverse plane movement in the foot. The forefoot adducts on the face-side leg, and the forefoot on the back leg abducts if it is still in a weight-bearing position.

The techniques in this chapter include most of the movements a baby practices in standing. Many of the techniques described in previous chapters also are preparatory movements to independent forward walking.

Do not rush into forward walking in your therapy sessions. Try to spend more time on the multiplaned preparatory movements, in a functional context, as babies typically do.

You can try the standing techniques with most of the babies with whom you work. The babies do not need full control in standing to practice these techniques because you will provide some of the support and control. However, for these facilitation techniques to be effective, the baby must participate actively in the process. The baby must know, share, and be interested in achieving the goal. You cannot **make** the baby walk; you only can facilitate how the baby walks.

The baby may need to wear orthotics during the facilitation, depending on the baby's mobility and control in the feet. If your facilitations proximally at the baby's hips can control the baby's feet, the baby does not need to wear orthotics during the facilitation. If you cannot control the baby's feet by what you do at the hips, the baby must wear orthotics during the facilitation.

12.1 Symmetrical Stance: Weight Shift to the Lateral Borders of the Feet

The goal of this facilitation is to activate the gluteus maximus in standing in order to extend the hips and transfer the weight to the lateral borders of the feet.

This technique is helpful for babies who stand with their weight on the medial sides of their feet (figure 12.1.1). With the weight distributed this way, the feet pronate and the femurs internally rotate.

Baby's Position The baby stands in front of you. The baby is usually more stable with the hands resting on a firm object. (The therapist did not use a surface in the photos so that the reader could see the various components of the baby's and the therapist's movements.)

Therapist's Position Sit or kneel behind the baby with your hands on the baby's femurs.

Therapist's Hands and Movement To control the baby's hips and knees, place your hands on the baby's femurs, just above the knees, fingers perpendicular around the femurs and thumbs across the hip joints or parallel to the femurs and pointing up toward the hips (figure 12.1.1). Parallel alignment of the thumbs is important for the facilitation of hip extension. Perpendicular placement of the thumbs across the femurs facilitates hip and knee flexion.

With your thumbs, subtly press in and up toward the hips, while your fingers simultaneously extend the baby's knees and provide a slight external rotation force to the femurs to activate the gluteus maximus. The external rotation must be sufficient to transfer the baby's weight to the lateral borders of the feet. In figures 12.1.2 and 12.1.3, the therapist has externally rotated the baby's left leg more than the right leg, and the weight has transferred to the lateral border of the left foot.

Take care not to produce knee hyperextension. This can occur if you use your fingers to pull the baby's knees into extension rather than using the subtle upward pressure of your thumbs to facilitate the extension.

If knee hyperextension does occur, reduce the backward force applied by your fingers, and apply a slight flexor force with the heels of your hands just above the baby's knees.

Precautions

- Pressure with the thumbs must not facilitate an anterior or posterior pelvic tilt. If either occurs, realign the thumbs on the gluteus maximus.
- Pressure with the thumbs must not facilitate ankle plantar flexion. If this occurs, use less upward pressure with your thumbs.

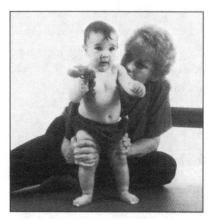

Figure 12.1.1. Symmetrical stance: Weight shift to the lateral borders of the feet. The therapist places her hands on the baby's femurs just above the knees, fingers perpendicular around the femurs and thumbs across the hip joints, parallel to the femurs, and pointing up toward the hips.

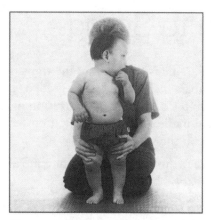

Figure 12.1.2. The therapist subtly presses in and up with her thumbs toward the hips, while her fingers simultaneously extend the baby's knees, provide a slight external rotation force to the femurs to activate the gluteus maximus, and transfer the baby's weight to the lateral borders of the feet.

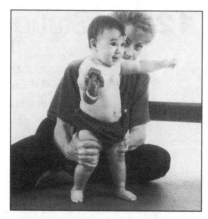

Figure 12.1.3. The therapist has externally rotated the baby's left leg more than the right leg, and the baby's weight has transferred to the lateral border of the left foot.

- Pressure with the thumbs must not facilitate knee hyperextension. If this occurs, a flexor counter pressure with the heels of the hands on the femurs will facilitate slight knee flexion.
- Backward pressure with the fingers must not facilitate knee hyperextension. If this occurs, reduce the backward pressure of the fingers.

Component Goals
- Hip and knee extension with ankle dorsiflexion
- Activation of the gluteus maximus and gluteus medius
- Transfer of weight to the lateral borders of the feet

Functional Goals
- Hip extensor control for all standing activities
- Gluteus maximus control for weight transference in the feet during gait

12.2 Standing to Sitting

The goal of this technique is to facilitate the transition from standing to sitting. Additional goals include increased graded eccentric control of the quadriceps and hip extensors with activation of the abdominals and activation of ankle dorsiflexors. This facilitation technique helps the baby learn to move on the sagittal plane.

The baby should use orthotics if you cannot control the baby's feet by your actions at the baby's hips.

Baby's Position The baby stands with hands resting on a firm object.

Therapist's Position Heel-sit behind the baby with your hands placed symmetrically on the baby's femurs.

Therapist's Hands and Movement Place your hands proximally on the baby's femurs. Spread your fingers so that your thumbs are on and can press into the baby's gluteus maximus and your little fingers are behind the baby's knee (figure 12.2.1). Your other fingers wrap around the baby's femurs. Your fourth finger may be behind the baby's knee or on the front of the femur, depending on the range of your finger spread.

To initiate the baby's transition to sitting, shift the baby's pelvis and weight slightly **backward** and down with both of your hands (figure 12.2.2). Flex the baby's hips and knees by carefully pressing your little fingers into the baby's knees. Maintain the pressure with your thumbs on the baby's gluteus maximus to control the eccentric activation of these muscles.

If it is difficult for you to use your little fingers, use the heels of your hands, rather than your little fingers, to press the baby's femurs forward and flex the knees as the baby's weight shifts **backward.**

Maintain the posterior weight shift and the flexed position of the baby's legs as you gradually lower the baby to sit on your legs (figure 12.2.3). If the baby has difficulty with range and/or eccentric control of knee flexion, you can raise your leg to meet the baby's hips.

The posterior weight shift should facilitate concentric activity in the baby's abdominals and ankle dorsiflexors and eccentric activity in the baby's quadriceps and gluteus maximus.

When the baby is sitting on your legs, continue to control the baby's lower-extremity posture (figure 12.2.4). Keep the knees flexed, the hips abducted, and the ankles at 90° dorsiflexion.

Try to keep the ankles at 90° rather than trying to increase the range of dorsiflexion by moving the tibia forward over the foot. You can facilitate the baby's ankle **dorsiflexor** muscles when you shift the baby's weight and center of mass backward and the ankles are at 90° with the weight on the heels of the baby's feet. Active dorsiflexion of the ankles elongates the gastrocnemius/soleus muscles.

If the tibia moves forward over the foot and greater dorsiflexion occurs, the gastrocnemius/soleus muscles may lengthen temporarily, but the

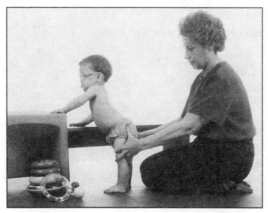

Figure 12.2.1. Standing to sitting. Kneel-sitting behind the standing baby, the therapist places her hands proximally on the baby's femurs, spreading her fingers so that the thumbs are on and can press into the baby's gluteus maximus and the fourth and fifth fingers are behind the baby's knee. The therapist's other fingers wrap around the baby's femurs.

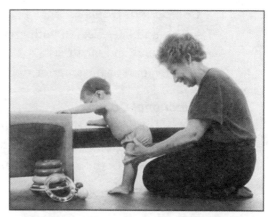

Figure 12.2.2. The therapist shifts the baby's pelvis and weight slightly backward and down with both hands, flexing the baby's hips and knees by carefully pressing her little fingers into the baby's knees. The therapist maintains the pressure with her thumbs on the baby's gluteus maximus to control the eccentric activation of these muscles.

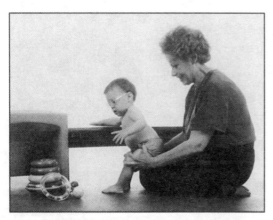

Figure 12.2.3. The therapist maintains the posterior weight shift and the flexed position of the baby's legs as she gradually lowers the baby to sit on her legs.

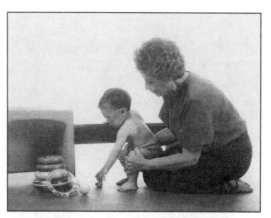

Figure 12.2.4. The therapist continues to control the baby's lower-extremity posture, keeping the baby's knees flexed, the hips abducted, and the ankles at 90° dorsiflexion.

forward weight shift transfers the weight and center of mass to the forefoot and actually facilitates ankle plantar flexion.

Suggestion Standing to sitting is a good technique to use for helping the baby retrieve toys that have dropped to the floor.

Precautions

- The baby's trunk must remain erect as the hips and knees flex.
- Shift the baby's hips posteriorly behind the feet.
- The ankles remain at 90°.
- Vary the height of your leg onto which the baby sits so the baby can practice different ranges of hip and knee flexion and eccentric gluteus maximus and quadriceps control.

Component Goals

- Hip and knee flexion with graded eccentric control in the gluteus maximus and quadriceps
- Activation of the anterior tibialis and abdominals

Functional Goals

- Graded eccentric control of the quadriceps and gluteus maximus for transitions from standing to sitting
- Activation of the anterior tibialis for use in gait

12.3 Lateral Weight Shift With Unilateral Hip Flexion

You may use this facilitation as a preparation for sideward cruising and/or climbing up stairs.

The goals of this facilitation are to learn how to transfer weight laterally when standing and to learn to control the posture in single-limb stance. Additional goals include activation of the gluteus maximus and medius with the trunk muscles, activation of the foot musculature in standing, and preparation for transference of weight to the lateral border of the feet during any standing activity. If you find it difficult to maintain the baby's weight on the lateral borders of the feet during these weight shifts, the baby should wear orthotics.

Baby's Position The baby stands in front of you, with the hands resting on a firm object.

Therapist's Position Kneel behind the baby with your hands on the lateral sides of the baby's femurs and knees.

Therapist's Hands and Movement Place your hands on the baby's femurs near or over the knees, fingers perpendicular around the femurs, thumbs parallel to the femurs pointing up toward the hips (figure 12.3.1).

Your *guiding hand* is on the soon-to-be weight-bearing leg (left leg in figure 12.3.1). Use your *guiding hand* to shift the baby's weight laterally. The weight shift must be sufficient to transfer the baby's weight to the lateral border of the (left) foot and to unweight the opposite (right) lower extremity.

If it is difficult for the baby to transfer the weight to the lateral border of the foot, externally rotate the femur with your fingers. When you do this, make sure you transfer the weight to the lateral border of the foot and that the entire leg does not rotate externally. The lateral weight shift must precede flexion of the unweighted leg.

Once the baby's weight has shifted laterally, flex the baby's unweighted (right) hip and knee forward with your *assisting hand* (figure 12.3.2). Initially, the baby may be able to tolerate only slight hip and knee flexion. As you practice this technique over time, gradually increase the degree of hip flexion. You may hold the leg in the air with the hip and knee flexed, or you may place the baby's foot on a small step positioned in front of the baby's feet.

The more hip flexion the baby can tolerate, the more the pelvis will be controlled on the sagittal plane. When the legs are in marked dissociation (as they are when one hip is in maximum flexion and the other hip is extended), the pelvis is not able to "fix" in an anterior or posterior pelvic tilt.

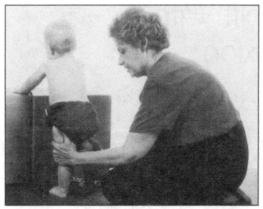

Figure 12.3.1. Lateral weight shift with unilateral hip flexion. The therapist places her hands on the baby's femurs near or over the knees, fingers perpendicular around the femurs, thumbs parallel to the femurs pointing up toward the hips. The therapist's *guiding (left) hand*, on the soon-to-be weight-bearing (left) leg, shifts the baby's weight laterally, transferring the baby's weight to the lateral border of the left foot and unweighting the right lower extremity.

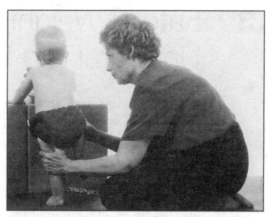

Figure 12.3.2. The therapist flexes the baby's unweighted (right) hip and knee forward with her *assisting (right) hand*.

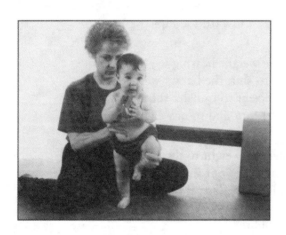

Figure 12.3.3. Front view. The therapist's *assisting (left) hand* flexes the baby's left leg. The therapist's *guiding (right) hand* is on the baby's trunk rather than on the baby's weight-bearing leg in order to stabilize the baby, because the baby does not have upper-extremity support. The therapist's *assisting hand* flexes the baby's left leg.

Figure 12.3.3 illustrates the position of the therapist's *assisting hand* on the baby's flexed leg.

Note: Because the baby does not have upper-extremity support, the therapist's *guiding hand* is on the baby's trunk rather than on the baby's weight-bearing leg in order to stabilize the baby.

Make sure you practice this technique on both sides and alternate from side to side, to emphasize the transition through midline.

Precautions

- You must transfer the baby's weight to and maintain the weight on the lateral border of the weight-bearing foot while the unweighted leg is flexed.

- Lift the baby's unweighted leg and flex it only after you have completed the weight shift successfully.
- Flex the baby's hip and knee as tolerated, but gradually work to increase the degree of flexion.

Component Goals

- Lateral weight shift of the body over the foot
- Transference of weight to the lateral border of the foot
- Activation of the gluteus maximus and gluteus medius
- Lower-extremity dissociation
- Control of the pelvis on the sagittal plane

Functional Goals

- Extension of the trunk, hip, and lower extremity to support the stance phase of gait
- Weight transference in the lower extremities needed for gait
- Flexion of the unweighted leg for stair climbing
- Postural and balance control necessary for single-limb stance, which is used in gait and stair climbing

12.4 Symmetrical Stance: Face-Side Rotation

The goals of this facilitation are to increase transverse plane mobility and control in the baby's trunk, pelvis, hips, and feet and to increase activation of the foot musculature.

If you find it difficult to transfer and/or maintain the baby's weight on the lateral borders of the feet during these weight shifts, the baby should wear orthotics.

Baby's Position The baby stands with hands resting on a firm object.

Therapist's Position Kneel behind the baby with your hands on the lateral sides of the baby's legs over the knees.

Therapist's Hands and Movement Place your hands on the baby's femurs, near or over the knees, fingers perpendicular around the femur and thumbs parallel to the femur, pointing up toward the hips (figures 12.4.1 through 12.4.4).

Your *guiding hand* is on the soon-to-be weight-bearing leg (right leg in figures 12.4.2 through 12.4.4). Your *guiding hand* externally rotates the baby's femur so that the baby's weight transfers to the lateral border of the foot (figures 12.4.2 and 12.4.4). This rotation is most effective when done in conjunction with the baby turning to see or reach for something in that direction (figure 12.4.4).

As the femur and lower leg externally rotate, the baby's weight-bearing foot assumes a position of slight inversion and adduction (figure 12.4.2, right foot).

Use your *assisting hand* to stabilize the less-weighted back leg in abduction with hip and knee extension (figure 12.4.2, left leg). Permit slight internal rotation of the leg. If possible, the foot of the back leg should continue to make contact with the floor. This foot moves toward eversion and abduction (figure 12.4.2, left foot).

Practice this technique for both sides, transitioning through midline.

Precautions
- Rotation must occur at the hip joint, not at the knee joint.
- The less-weighted back leg moves into **slight** internal rotation. Do not let the leg drop into marked internal rotation.
- You must maintain the less-weighted back leg in abduction with hip and knee extension. Do not let the leg drop into adduction with hip and knee flexion.

Component Goals
- Rotational weight shift of the body over the foot
- Pelvic-femoral (hip joint) mobility and control
- Balance reactions in the unweighted leg of hip extension, abduction, and slight internal rotation

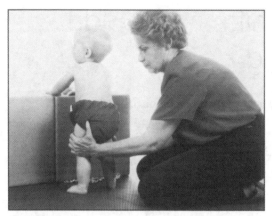

Figure 12.4.1. Symmetrical stance: Face-side rotation. The therapist places her hands on the baby's femurs, over the knees, fingers perpendicular around the femur and thumbs parallel to the femur, pointing up toward the hips.

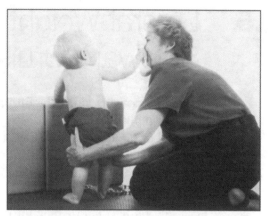

Figure 12.4.2. The therapist's *guiding (right) hand*, on the soon-to-be weight-bearing (right) leg, externally rotates the baby's femur so that the baby's weight transfers to the lateral border of the foot. As the femur and lower leg externally rotate, the baby's weight-bearing foot assumes a position of slight inversion and adduction. The therapist's *assisting (left) hand* stabilizes the less-weighted back leg in abduction with hip and knee extension.

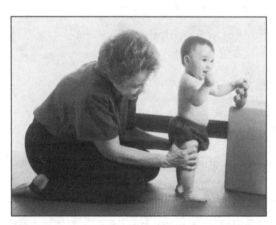

Figure 12.4.3. Side view of therapist's hand position for externally rotating the baby's right leg.

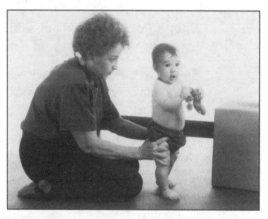

Figure 12.4.4. The therapist's *guiding (right) hand* externally rotates the baby's right femur so that the baby's weight transfers to the lateral border of the foot. The therapist's *assisting (left) hand* stabilizes the baby's left leg in abduction with hip and knee extension. The baby's turning to the right enhances the facilitation.

Functional Goals

- Rotational weight shift control, used in gait
- Preparation for midstance control of the weighted lower extremity
- Equilibrium reactions with extension and rotation in standing
- Extension of the unweighted leg, used in terminal stance

12.5 Lateral Weight Shifts: Sideward Cruising

Sideward cruising along the furniture is the baby's first means of upright mobility. Sideward cruising helps the baby develop frontal plane control of the lower extremities, trunk, and even upper-extremity muscles. Sideward cruising helps the baby learn how to transfer the weight laterally to one leg so the other leg can move.

It is important that you spend a lot of time on the baby's sideward cruising rather than rushing into forward walking. Many of the foundational components of forward walking develop in cruising. As the baby practices cruising, the lateral movements gradually incorporate rotation (transverse plane movement). As the baby continually adds more rotation, the sideward stepping transitions to forward stepping.

The goals of this facilitation are activation of the gluteus maximus and medius with the trunk muscles, activation of the foot musculature in standing, and preparation for transference of weight to the lateral border of the feet during any standing activity. If you find it difficult to maintain the baby's weight on the lateral borders of the feet during these weight shifts, the baby should wear orthotics.

Baby's Position The baby stands in front of you, with the hands resting on a firm object.

Therapist's Position Kneel behind the baby in a position that permits you to move with the baby.

Therapist's Hands Place your hands on the baby's femurs, above or over the knees, fingers perpendicular around the femur, thumbs on the gluteus maximus or parallel to the femur and pointing up toward the hips (figure 12.5.1).

The *guiding hand* is on the soon-to-be weight-bearing leg. If the baby is cruising to the left, the first weight shift is to the right leg (figure 12.5.2). The *assisting hand* is on the soon-to-be unweighted leg. The lateral weight shift to the right leg must precede abduction of the left leg.

Movement The *guiding hand* shifts the baby's weight laterally (to the right in figure 12.5.2) sufficiently to unweight the opposite (left) lower extremity. The lateral weight shift to the right must precede abduction of the left leg.

Transfer the weight to the lateral border of the baby's (right) foot. If it is difficult for the baby to transfer the weight to the lateral border, externally rotate the femur with your fingers. When you externally rotate the femur, make sure that the weight transfers to the lateral border of the foot and that the entire leg does not rotate externally.

Once the baby's weight has shifted, abduct the baby's unweighted (left) leg with your *assisting hand* while maintaining the hip and knee in extension (figure 12.5.2). If the knee tends to flex, place your hand over

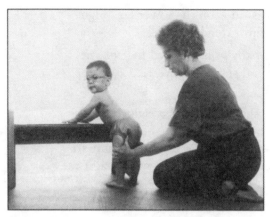

Figure 12.5.1. Lateral weight shifts: Sideward cruising. The therapist places her hands on the baby's femurs over the knees, fingers perpendicular around the femur, thumbs on the gluteus maximus parallel to the femur and pointing up toward the hips.

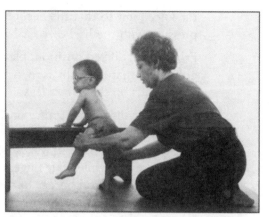

Figure 12.5.2. The therapist's *guiding (right) hand*, on the weight-bearing (right) leg, shifts the baby's weight laterally to the right sufficiently to unweight the left lower extremity. The lateral weight shift to the right precedes abduction of the left leg. The therapist abducts the baby's unweighted (left) leg with her *assisting hand* while maintaining the hip and knee in extension.

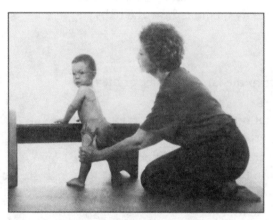

Figure 12.5.3. Keeping her hands on the baby's legs, the therapist places the baby's unweighted (left) foot on the ground so that the baby is in symmetrical stance.

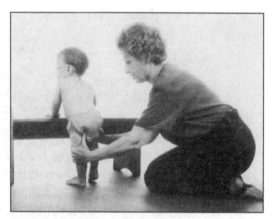

Figure 12.5.4. From the symmetrical stance position, the therapist shifts the baby's weight laterally to the left foot as her *assisting (left) hand* helps stabilize the hip and knee extension. She presses up toward the hip with her thumb to extend the hip while her fingers externally rotate the femur to shift the weight to the lateral border of the foot. The therapist's *guiding (right) hand* unweights and abducts the baby's right leg, then adducts it so that the baby is once again in double-limb stance.

the knee joint so that the heel of your hand is on the lower leg. Slight pressure with the heel of your hand helps extend the knee.

From the abducted position, place the baby's unweighted foot on the ground so that the baby is in symmetrical stance (figure 12.5.3). Keep your hands on the baby's legs.

From the symmetrical stance position, shift the baby's weight laterally to the left foot as your *assisting hand* helps stabilize the hip and knee extension (figure 12.5.4). Press up toward the hip with your thumb to extend the hip while your fingers externally rotate the femur to shift the weight to the lateral border of the foot.

After you shift the baby's weight to the second (left) leg, unweight and abduct the baby's first (right) leg with your *guiding hand* (figure 12.5.4), then adduct it so that the baby is once again in double-limb stance. From double-limb stance, repeat the procedure.

It is important to practice this technique in both directions so that all of the hip muscles have the opportunity to contract both concentrically and eccentrically.

For this facilitation to be effective, the baby must participate actively in the process. The baby must know and share the goal (e.g., to get the toy at the end of the bench) and be interested in achieving the goal. You **cannot make** the baby cruise; you can only facilitate **how** the baby cruises.

Precautions

- You must maintain the weight shift to the lateral border of the foot while you abduct the unweighted leg.
- You must maintain the baby's weight on the lateral border of the foot for the hip and knee to respond appropriately.
- Abduct the unweighted leg in a short range. If the abduction is too great, the baby will have difficulty shifting weight onto that leg.
- When you place the unweighted foot on the floor, you must transfer the weight to the lateral border of the foot.

Component Goals

- Frontal plane control of the trunk, hips, and feet
- Lateral weight shift of the body over the foot
- Transference of weight to the lateral border of the foot
- Eccentric activation of the hip abductors and concentric activation of the hip adductor muscles on the stance leg
- Activation of the gluteus maximus
- Concentric activation of the hip abductors on the unweighted leg

Functional Goals

- Lateral weight shifts for cruising around the furniture
- Preparatory activities for forward gait

12.6 Facilitation From the Rib Cage and Pelvis: Sagittal Plane Control

The goal of this facilitation is to align and maintain the alignment of the baby's trunk and pelvis on the sagittal plane during forward ambulation.

If the baby has an anterior or posterior pelvic tilt, your hands work synchronously to align the baby's ribs, pelvis, and hips to neutral on the sagittal plane (figure 12.6.1).

Baby's Position The baby stands sideways to you. The baby's hands are free at the sides, or the shoulders may flex forward to push a firm object.

Forward flexion of the arms helps transfer the weight posteriorly to the heels and helps activate the anterior trunk muscles. Retraction of the arms and shoulder girdles causes the weight to transfer to the balls of the feet, resulting in ankle plantar flexion and activation of the posterior trunk muscles.

Therapist's Position Kneel on the floor or sit on a mobile stool beside the baby. You must be in a position to move with the baby.

Therapist's Hands and Movement Place your *guiding hand* on the baby's lower anterior rib cage and abdominals and lightly press down and in to align the rib cage with the pelvis (figures 12.6.1 and 12.6.2). Do not push the trunk into flexion or the pelvis into a posterior pelvic tilt.

Place your *assisting hand* on the baby's gluteus maximus across both hip joints (not across the sacrum) to facilitate hip extension (figure 12.6.1). Place the fingers of your hand on one gluteus maximus and the thumb or the heel of your hand on the other gluteus maximus. Press in and down with your hand.

With the rib cage and pelvis aligned, the baby will not need to retract the shoulder girdles for trunk stability (figures 12.6.1, 12.6.2).

While keeping the rib cage-pelvic alignment, use your *guiding hand* together with your *assisting hand* and carefully shift the baby's weight laterally onto one (right) leg (figure 12.6.1). This unweights the baby's other (left) leg and frees it to move forward (figure 12.6.2). Once the baby's (left) leg has advanced forward, use your hands to shift the baby's weight laterally and slightly forward to the forward (left) leg. This unweights the back (right) leg and frees it to advance forward (figure 12.6.3).

Maintain the baby's neutral rib cage-pelvic alignment with your hands as the baby walks forward. The baby's arms are free to swing reciprocally with the legs. You will feel the baby's abdominals and hip extensors contract as the baby walks. It is the baby's active lower-extremity movements that activate the abdominal and hip muscles, not your hands; your hands maintain the alignment.

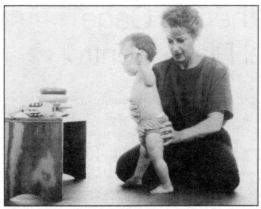

Figure 12.6.1. Facilitation from the rib cage and pelvis: Sagittal plane control. The therapist places her *guiding (right) hand* on the baby's lower anterior rib cage and abdominals and presses down and in lightly to align the rib cage with the pelvis. The *assisting (left) hand* is on the baby's gluteus maximus across both hip joints (fingers on one gluteus maximus and thumb on the other gluteus maximus) to facilitate hip extension. Keeping the rib cage-pelvic alignment, the therapist uses her *guiding hand* together with the *assisting hand* to shift the baby's weight laterally onto the baby's right leg.

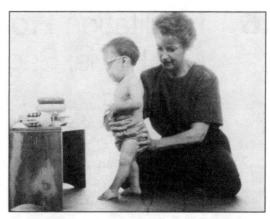

Figure 12.6.2. Counterrotation. The baby's weight shifts to the right leg, and the fingers of the therapist's *guiding hand* rotate the left side of the baby's rib cage back as the baby's left unweighted leg swings forward.

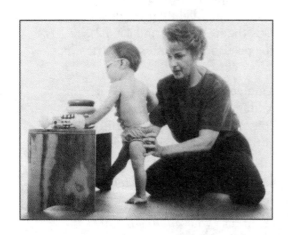

Figure 12.6.3. Counterrotation. The therapist's hands shift the baby's weight to the left leg. The heel of the therapist's *guiding hand* rotates the right side of the baby's rib cage back as the baby's right leg swings forward.

Counterrotation

Counterrotation is the reciprocal rotation of the upper and lower trunk. When the right side of the pelvis rotates forward, the right side of the rib cage rotates backward. Counterrotation in the trunk is synchronous with reciprocal movements of the upper and lower extremities. When the right leg swings forward, the right arm swings backward.

If the baby has difficulty with counterrotation during forward walking, you can facilitate counterrotation with the hand placement described on page 237. Your *guiding hand* facilitates rib cage rotation while your *assisting hand* maintains the hip extension. Your *guiding hand* rotates the ribs back on the side of the swing leg.

In figures 12.6.1 and 12.6.2, the baby's weight shifts to the right leg, and the fingers of the therapist's *guiding hand* rotate the left side of the baby's rib cage back as the baby's left leg swings forward (figure 12.6.2). In figure 12.6.3, the baby's weight shifts to the left leg, and the heel of the therapist's *guiding hand* rotates the right side of the baby's rib cage back as the baby's right leg swings forward.

Your *assisting hand* on the baby's gluteus maximus helps the baby maintain hip extension on the weight-bearing leg as the weight shifts to that leg and the opposite leg swings forward. If the baby's hip is unstable during the lateral weight shift, apply increased pressure to the hip extensors with your *assisting hand* to increase the stability of the hip.

Do not rotate the pelvis with your *assisting hand*. The forward swing of the baby's unweighted leg produces subtle, but sufficient, forward rotation of the pelvis on that side.

Precautions

- Do not cause a posterior pelvic tilt by excessive pushing on the baby's lower ribs.
- Do not cause hip hyperextension or an anterior pelvic tilt by pushing the baby's hips too far forward.
- Do not place your hand on the baby's sacrum or lumbar spine; this produces an anterior pelvic tilt and hip flexion.
- Be careful to rotate the **ribs** back on the side of the swing leg.
- Do not rotate the pelvis.

Component Goals

- Alignment of the rib cage over the pelvis
- Neutral pelvic tilt
- Hip extension with synergistic oblique abdominal activity
- Controlled lateral weight shifts of the trunk and pelvis over the femur and the foot
- Counterrotation of the upper trunk over the lower trunk
- Reciprocal arm swing

Functional Goals

- Forward walking with sagittal plane neutral alignment of the ribs, pelvis, and hips
- Preparation for active arm swinging with independent ambulation

12.7 Facilitation From the Rib Cage and Pelvis: Frontal Plane Control

The goal of this facilitation is to align and maintain the alignment of the baby's trunk and pelvis on the frontal plane during forward ambulation.

If the baby has lateral shifting, leaning of the rib cage, and/or poor hip abductor control, your hands work synchronously to align the baby's ribs, pelvis, and hips to neutral on the frontal plane (figure 12.7.1).

Baby's Position The baby stands in front of you. The baby's hands are free at the sides, or the shoulders may flex forward to push a firm object.

Therapist's Position Kneel or sit on a mobile stool behind the baby, in a position to move with the baby. Place your hands on the lateral aspect of the baby's ribs, pelvis, and hips.

Therapist's Hands and Movement Both hands work together to stabilize the baby's rib cage-pelvic-hip alignment and to assist with lateral weight shifts. The index finger on each hand works alternately to facilitate rib cage rotation.

Place your hands laterally on the baby's trunk so that the palms of your hands are on the baby's pelvis and hip joints, your thumbs are on the back of the pelvis, and your index fingers are on the lateral sides of the rib cage. Your other three fingers abduct and spread to reach to the baby's lateral abdominals and femurs (figures 12.7.1 and 12.7.2). Do not place your fingers on the hip flexors.

Push in and down with your hands to stabilize the baby's trunk, pelvis, and hips (figures 12.7.1 and 12.7.2). In this technique, your hands stabilize the rib cage-pelvic-hip alignment as the baby walks forward.

If baby has difficulty with lateral weight shifts, your hands help facilitate the weight shift. The weight shift must occur with the trunk and pelvis moving as a unit over the stance leg. The rib cage must not lean nor shift laterally over the pelvis. The pelvis must stay in line with the femur.

Counterrotation

If the baby has difficulty with counterrotation of the rib cage over the pelvis, facilitate the counterrotation with your index fingers. Your hands and points of stability remain the same.

Facilitate counterrotation by providing a slight backward pressure with your index finger on the baby's ribs on the side of the swing leg, while both of your thumbs stabilize the baby's pelvis.

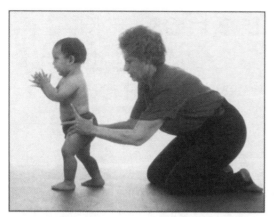

Figure 12.7.1. Facilitation from the rib cage and pelvis: Frontal plane control. The therapist places her hands laterally on the baby's trunk so that the palms of her hands are on the baby's pelvis and hip joints, her thumbs are on the back of the pelvis, and her index fingers are on the lateral sides of the rib cage. Her other three fingers abduct and spread to reach to the baby's lateral abdominals and femurs.

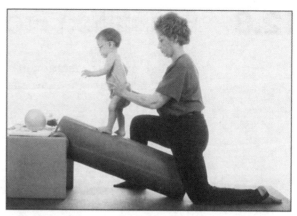

Figure 12.7.2. The therapist pushes in and down with her hands to stabilize the baby's trunk, pelvis, and hips as the baby walks forward on an inclined bolster.

When the baby's weight is on the left leg and the right leg is in swing, provide slight backward pressure to the right side of the baby's ribs with your right index finger. Both of your thumbs stabilize the baby's pelvis.

When the baby's weight is on the right leg and the left leg is in swing, provide slight backward pressure to the left side of the baby's ribs with your left index finger. Both of your thumbs stabilize the baby's pelvis.

Alternate your hand movements as the baby walks forward.

Suggestion To provide variety and motivation for the baby, use an inclined bolster (figure 12.7.2). Stabilize the bolster with a cube chair.

Component Goals

- Rib cage-pelvic-hip alignment on the frontal plane during gait
- Counterrotation of the rib cage and pelvis during gait
- Reciprocal arm swing

Functional Goals

- Counterrotation of the upper and lower trunk during gait
- Reciprocal arm swing

12.8 Facilitation From the Hips

The goals of this facilitation are to help the baby align the pelvis and femurs and control the movements of the lower extremities during ambulation.

The baby should wear orthotics if you cannot control the baby's feet by what you do at the femurs.

Baby's Position The baby stands in front of you. The baby's hands are free at the sides, or the shoulders may flex forward to push a firm object.

Therapist's Position Kneel or sit on a mobile stool behind the baby, in a position to move with the baby.

Therapist's Hands and Movement Place your hands over the lateral aspect of the baby's hip joints, across the hip abductor muscles. Wrap your fingers around the baby's femurs and place your thumbs on the baby's gluteus maximus (figures 12.8.1 and 12.8.2). Press your hands in and down to stabilize the baby's hip joints. Both hands will maintain this placement throughout the facilitation.

Your *guiding hand* is on the soon-to-be weight-bearing leg. You will use your thumbs to facilitate the baby's hip extensors; your fingers will apply downward pressure on the leg into the foot and rotate the femur externally. Each hand alternately becomes the *guiding hand*.

Your *assisting hand* has the same placement as the *guiding hand*.

Your hands work together to facilitate a lateral weight shift of the baby's pelvis and trunk over one leg. As the baby's weight shifts to one leg, the thumb of your *guiding hand* simultaneously presses into the baby's gluteus maximus to facilitate hip extension and subtle forward movement of the pelvis.

When the baby's weight shifts laterally, the weight should transfer to the lateral border of the foot. If the baby has difficulty transferring the weight to the lateral border of the foot, use the fingers of your *guiding hand* to rotate the baby's femur externally. When the baby's foot is in a weight-bearing position and the knee is extended, external rotation of the femur facilitates external rotation of the tibia, which subsequently transfers the weight to the lateral border of the foot.

Once the baby's weight has shifted, your *guiding hand* maintains the extension and lateral weight shift on the weight-bearing leg as the baby swings the unweighted leg forward and places the foot on the floor (figures 12.8.1 and 12.8.3).

If the baby has difficulty swinging the unweighted leg forward, keep your hands on the hips, but place the little finger of your *assisting hand* behind the baby's unweighted femur, and guide it forward until the foot is on the floor.

Once the foot is on the floor, maintain the baby's back leg in extension with your *guiding hand* and shift the baby's weight onto the forward

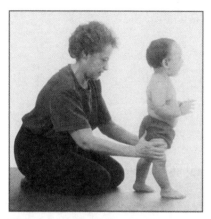

Figure 12.8.1. Facilitation from the hips. The therapist's *guiding hand* is on the soon-to-be weight-bearing (right) leg. As both hands work together to facilitate a lateral weight shift of the baby's pelvis and trunk over the right leg, the guiding-hand thumb presses into the baby's right gluteus maximus to facilitate hip extension and subtle forward movement of the pelvis.

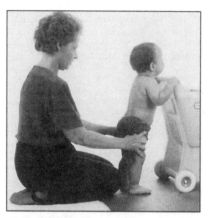

Figure 12.8.2. Pushing a cart to facilitate shoulder flexion. The therapist places her hands over the lateral aspects of the baby's hip joints and across the hip abductor muscles, wrapping her fingers around the baby's femurs and placing her thumbs on the baby's gluteus maximus. The therapist presses her hands in and down to stabilize the baby's hip joints.

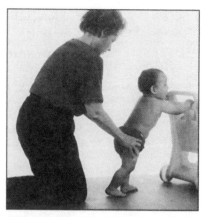

Figure 12.8.3. Once the baby's left foot is on the floor, the therapist maintains the baby's right leg in extension with her *guiding hand* as she shifts the baby's weight onto the forward (left) leg. As the baby's right leg becomes more extended, the baby's weight rolls over the toes of the back foot and the leg moves into a terminal-stance position.

leg (figures 12.8.1 and 12.8.3). As the baby's back leg becomes more extended, the baby's weight rolls over the toes of the back foot into a terminal stance position (figure 12.8.3), which elongates the hip flexors, toe flexors, and plantar fascia.

Suggestion Use a baby cart to motivate the baby to walk forward and to facilitate active shoulder flexion (figure 12.8.3).

Precautions

- You must maintain the lateral weight shift and hip extension on the stance leg while the unweighted leg swings forward.
- The baby must participate actively with the hip flexion and knee extension of the swing leg.
- Do not place your hands on the baby's iliac crest or pelvis above the hip joint. If your hands are above the hip joint, the baby will not have hip joint stability.

Component Goals

- Lateral weight shift of the body over the foot
- Dynamic control of the pelvic-femoral (hip joint) muscles during lateral weight shift in stance
- Transference of weight toward the lateral border of the foot
- Activation of the gluteus maximus and gluteus medius on the stance leg
- Eccentric hip abductor control in gait
- Active hip flexion on the swing leg

- Elongation of the hip flexors, toe flexors, and plantar fascia on the back leg
- Lower-extremity dissociation

Functional Goals
- Forward walking
- Controlled lateral weight shift of the trunk and pelvis over the stance leg during gait
- Hip, knee, ankle, and toe extension, used in the terminal stance phase of gait
- Pushing an object while walking

Index

A

accommodation of the hand, 153
activation of abdominal muscles, 19–23, 92, 226–228
    over bolster, 104–107
    oblique, 28–30, 154, 161–163, 200–202
    in prone straddle, 94–95
    in sidelying, 39, 102–103
    in transition to standing, 134–135
    in walking, 237–239
activation of anterior tibialis, 226–228
activation of elbow extensors, 139–140
activation of extensors, 187–188
    and flexors, 190–192, 204
activation of eye muscles, 13, 19–23
activation of flexors, 186–187
    and extensors, 190–192, 204
activation of foot musculature, 229–231, 232–233, 234–236
activation of gluteus maximus, 97–98, 122, 132, 210, 224–225
    eccentric, 226
    and gluteus medius, 229–231, 234–236, 241–243
activation of head flexors, 56–60
    and extensors, 190–192
activation of head, neck, and trunk flexors, 11–13, 14–18, 19–23, 24–27
activation of hip extensors, 47–49, 132
    and climbing, 113–114
    and flexors, 203–205
    and lateral weight shift, 50–52
    in transition from prone, 117–120
activation of hip flexors, 56–60, 187, 203–205
activation of lower trapezius muscles, 19, 66
activation of muscles on unweighted side, 56–60
activation of neck flexors, 42–45, 56–60
activation of neck and trunk extensors, 37–40, 43–44
    coactivation with flexors, 200–202, 203–206
    prone on lap, 47–49
activation of neck and trunk flexors, 31–33, 37–40, 43
    coactivation with extensors, 200–202, 203–206
    with shoulder flexors, 34–46
activation of neck muscles, 11–14, 22, 31–33, 34, 39–40
    and lateral weight shift, 50–52
    in 6-month roll, 42–45
activation of pectoral muscles, 81–82, 87–89, 90–92, 200–202
    in sidelying, 83–86
activation of serratus anterior, 81–82, 83–86
activation of shoulder girdle muscles, 70–73, 81–82, 83–86
    in prone straddle, 94–95
    in runner's stretch, 90–93
activation of trunk extensors, 37–40, 47–49, 193–198
    and flexors, 190–192, 200–202, 203–205
    and lateral weight shift, 50–52
    in 6-month roll, 42–45
    in transition from prone, 117–120

activation of trunk flexors, 42–45, 56–60
activation of trunk muscles, 31–33, 34–36, 117–120, 237–239
    diagonal, 161–163
    in runner's stretch, 90–93
active chin tuck, 185–187
active head/neck rotation, 19–23, 157–160
active reaching. *See:* reaching
age-appropriateness, 5, 7, 19
"air standing," 187–188
alert state, 2, 183, 186
ambulation, 237–239, 240–241, 242–244.
    See also: walking
ankle dorsiflexion, 129–131, 132–133, 178–181, 226–228
ankle joint mobility, 106
ankle plantar flexion, 132–134, 178–181, 224, 227, 237
    transition to dorsiflexion, 132–138
anterior weight shift, 40
    for activation of extensors, 187–188
    over ball, 65–67
    on bolster, 209–214, 216–218
    and hip joint mobility, 209–214
    in quadruped, 124–126
    response to, 185–189, 203–205
    in rising to stand, 169–170
    and 6-month roll, 43–44
assisting hand, 7
attention system, 2
auditory system, 35
autonomic system, 1, 2

B

backward weight shift. *See:* posterior weight shift
balance reactions, 103,141–143, 152–156
    with extension and rotation, 193–198
    in sitting, 139–140, 200–202
    in symmetrical stance, 205–206, 232–233
balance: in half-kneeling, 178–181, 215–218
    in standing, 213–214, 229–231
ball, 8
    bouncing on, 183–184
    prone on, 74–77, 78–80
    and reaching, 139–140
    rotation with flexion on, 200–202
    selection of, 68, 185
    in transition to sitting, 58–59
    and weight bearing, 70–73
    weight shift over, 65–67
bear standing, 113–115, 118–119
behavioral language, 1, 2
behavioral state, regulation of, 1
biomechanics, of cerebral palsy, 4–5
bite reflex, 14–18
body exploration, 7, 14–18, 85, 152–153
    with hands and eyes, 24–27
    in sidelying, 53–55, 83–86

F

face-side rotation, 232–233
facilitation technique, xvii, 6–7
family members, 8
feedforward, 3
feet, pronation of, 5, 68, 224.
    See also: lateral borders of feet, lower-extremity weight
        bearing
finger fisting, 18
five-month position, 38–40, 128–131
five-month roll. *See:* rolling
Floor Transitions, 117–138
    long-sit to quadruped with forward vaulting, 124–127
    long-sit to 5-month position, 128–131
    prone to lower-extremity dissociation, 117–120
    prone to standing, 132–138
    sitting to quadruped to kneeling, 121–123
forearm weight bearing, 70–73, 81 82, 83–86, 90–91
    in 6-month roll, 42–45.
    See also: upper-extremity weight bearing
forward protective extension reaction, 65–67, 97–99,
    139–140
forward vaulting, 124–127
four-month roll. *See:* rolling
frontal plane, 4, 223, 234–236, 240–241

G

gait cycle, 173–177
    and counterrotation, 240–241
    hip control and, 242–244
    midstance position of, 166, 167, 169, 171, 199
    preparation for, 128–131, 222, 225, 229–231, 234–236
    push-off, 117–120
    rotational weight shift control of, 233
    swing position of, 166, 169, 171
    terminal stance of, 117, 233, 242–244
gastrostomy tube, 47
grasp reflex, 17–18, 24–27
grasping, 24–27, 53–55, 70–73
guiding hand, 7

H

half-kneeling, 106, 119–120, 132–138, 215–218
    rotation to, 178–181
hand: arches in, 94–95
    to arms, 15, 16
    to face, 16–17
    to feet, 26, 31–33, 53–55, 83–84
    to hand, 17, 24
    to head, 17
    to hips, 21
    to knees, 25, 34–36, 37–40
    to legs, 25–26
    to mouth, 17
    and play, 83–86, 97–99
    and tactile exploration, 14–18
hand shaping, 14–18, 19–23, 152–153
"happy face" technique, 141–143, 148–151
head: activation of, 11–13
    control of, 23

extension of, 56–60
lateral flexion of, 18, 22, 75–76, 83–86
lifting, 47–49, 50–52, 90–92
lateral righting, 28–29, 61–64, 70–73, 74–77, 83–86
rotation, 19–23, 34, 61–64, 78–80, 94–95
in rolling, 31–33
and sensory input, 3
head, trunk, and hip extension, 56–60, 173–177
head and trunk flexion, 34–36, 37–41, 42–45, 83–86, 87–89
hip and knee extension, 42–45
    over ball, 65–69
    over bolster, 100–103, 104–107
    in cruising, 234–236
    in 5-month position, 128–131
    in floor transitions, 117–120
    in preparation for standing, 65–69
    in prone straddle, 94–95
    in rising to stand, 166–167, 169–172, 173–177
    in rotation to stand, 198
    in runner's stretch, 90–93
hip extension, 74, 76, 78–80, 87–89
    in ambulation, 237–239, 242–244
    in bear standing, 113–115
    over bolster, 97–99, 100–103, 104–107, 215–218
    in cruising, 234–236
    difficulty with, 187, 205
    in 5-month roll, 37–41
    in half-kneeling, 178–181, 215–218
    with knee flexion, 132–138
    and one-leg stand, 198–199
    in prone straddle, 94–95
    in rising to stand, 166–167, 170–171, 211, 219–222
    with rotation, 61–64, 194–195
    in runner's stretch, 92
    in standing, 213, 224–225, 232–233
    symmetrical, 97–99
    and transition to prone, 117–120
    with trunk extension, 121–123
hip flexion, 21, 74–77, 117–120, 215–218, 243
    with abduction and external rotation, 154–156, 178–181
    in climbing, 108
    in 5-month roll, 37–41
    in lateral weight shift, 50–52
    prone on lap, 47–49
    in runner's stretch, 90–91
    in transition to standing, 132–138, 229–231
hip hyperextension, 239
hip joints, 157–160, 209–214
hip mobility, 157–160, 161–163, 165–168
    in half-kneeling, 178–181, 215–218
    in transition to standing, 169–172, 173–177, 209–214.
    See also: pelvic-femoral mobility
humerus, 16–17, 29, 207–208
hypermobility, 124, 174, 209, 215
hypertonia, 2
hypotonia, 2, 127, 209

I, J, K

kinesiological issues, xv, 4–5
kinesthetic system, 3

knee extension, 74–77, 173–177, 215–218, 234–236
    over bolster, 100–103, 104–107
    difficulty with, 198
    in 5-month roll, 37–41
    prone on ball, 65–69
    in prone straddle, 94–95
    in rising to stand, 166–167, 170–171
    with rotation, 61–64
    in runner's stretch, 90–93
    in standing, 220, 232–233
knee, 215–218, 224–225
kneeling, 121–123, 133–134
Kong, Elsbeth, iii, vii
kyphosis, 4–5, 8, 209

L
lateral borders of feet, 5
    cruising and, 234–236
    in single-limb stance, 221
    in standing from bolster, 212
    and walking, 242
    weight shift to, 68–69, 224–225, 229–231, 232–233
lateral righting reactions, 28–30, 132–138
    of head and trunk, 53–55, 70–73, 81–82, 83–86, 90–93,
        141–143, 190–192
    with lateral weight shifts, 50–52, 53–55, 70–73, 74–77,
        91–92, 144–147, 148–151
    in movement to sitting, 56–60, 87–89
    in sidelying, 37–41, 100–103
    in symmetrical rolling, 31–33, 34–36
lateral weight shift, 74–77
    for activating flexors and extensors, 190–192
    in ambulation, 237–239, 240–241, 242–244
    and bear standing, 113–115
    and cruising, 234–236
    with elongation of scapulo-humeral muscles, 144–147
    with elongation of weight–bearing side, 132–138
    and "happy face" technique, 141–143, 148–151
    in prone, 50–52
    in runner's stretch, 90–91
    in sidelying, 104–107
    in standing, 213–214, 223
    with unilateral hip flexion, 229–231
    in upper extremities, 53–55, 70–73, 94–95
latissimus dorsi, 47–49, 50–52, 56–60, 83–86, 100–103
    with lateral righting, 144–147, 151
ligamentous laxity, 75–77
lordosis, 94, 209
lower-extremity dissociation, 100–103, 104–107
    in asymmetrical roll, 42–45
    on bolster, 215–218
    and carrying, 53–55
    and climbing, 108–112
    and diagonal weight shift, 157–160
    in 5-month position, 128–131
    in 5-month roll, 37–41
    with lateral weight shift, 229–231
    preparation for, 56–60
    in prone, 50–52
    in rising to stand, 132–138, 169–172

in rotation to half-kneeling, 178–181
in rotation to stand, 165–168, 173–177
in runner's stretch, 90–93
in sidelying, 83–86
in transition from prone, 117–120
in transition to sitting, 87–89
in walking, 242–244
lower-extremity mobility, 53–55, 100–103, 104–107,
    157–160
    and 5-month position, 128–131
    in half-kneeling, 215–218
    for walking, 161–163
lower-extremity weight bearing: in bear–standing, 113
    on both legs, 232–233, 237
    in 5-month position, 128–131
    on knee, 178–181, 215–218
    on leg and knee, 135–137
    single-limb, 102–103, 105, 125, 167, 169–171, 198–199,
        220–222, 229–231
    for sideward cruising, 234–236
    for standing and walking, 68–69, 173–177, 187–188,
        203–206.
    See also: single-limb stance, standing
lumbar flexion, 207, 209–210
lumbar hyperextension, 209, 212

M, N, O
midstance position. See: gait cycle
milestones, 5
motor impairments, 3, 185, 203
motor system, 1, 2
movement disorders, 209
musculoskeletal system, 4
music, 7
neutral alignment of hips, 66–67, 68–69
neutral alignment of trunk and pelvis, 187–188, 190–191,
    193–194, 237–239, 240–241
    in sitting, 200–202
one-leg stand. See: single-limb stance
orthotics, 5, 68, 223, 229, 232, 242

P
past-present-future order, 5–6
peanut ball, 102, 106–107, 139–140, 193–199
pelvic mobility, 161–163, 165–168
    in transition to standing, 157–160, 169–172, 173–177
pelvic rotation, 109–112
pelvic tilt, 224, 229, 237, 239
    anterior, 94, 209, 211–212
    posterior, 207
pelvic-femoral control, 242–244
pelvic-femoral (hip joint) mobility, 87–89, 105–106
    in anterior weight shifts, 209–214
    in diagonal weight shifts, 157–159,161–163, 193–199
    in half-kneeling, 178–181, 215–218
    in lateral weight shifts, 190–192
    in rising to stand, 165–168
    and single-limb stance, 198–199, 220–221
    in symmetrical stance, 232–233
planes of movement, 4, 5

plantar fascia, 243
play, 7
    with body, 14–18, 24–27, 152
    over bolster, 97–99
    in bouncing, 183–184
    in elongated side-sitting, 106–107
    on floor, 117
    preparation for, 53–55
    in sidelying, 37–41
    in sitting, 207
    to encourage turning, 158, 162, 197
    with one hand, 81–82, 83–86.
    See also: toys
posterior weight shift: for activation of flexors, 186
    over ball, 68–69
    and 5-month roll, 39–40, 43
    in half-kneeling, 216, 218
    in quadruped, 122
    response to, 185–189, 203–205
    in rising to stand, 170–171
    in single-limb stance, 221
    in standing, 167
    in transition to sitting, 226–228
postural adjustments, 3, 78–80
    and balance, 103
    and lateral righting, 141–143
postural control, 161–163, 183–184, 229–231
    in sitting, 207–208
pronation. *See:* feet
Prone on Ball, 65–80
    lateral righting reactions and sideways protective
        extension, 74–77
    prone extension: forward weight shift for trunk and hip
        extension and forward protective extension, 65–69
    prone to sit on the ball, 78–80
    upper-extremity weight bearing and weight shifts, 70–73
Prone on Bolster, 97–115
    climbing: bear standing, 113–115
    climbing: quadruped, 108–112
    prone to sidelying with lower-extremity dissociation,
        100–103
    prone to sidelying with lower-extremity weight-bearing
        progression, 104–107
    sitting to prone on bolster: symmetrical hip extension,
        97–99
Prone on Floor, 81–95
    prone straddle, 94–95
    prone to runner's stretch position, 90–93
    prone to sitting, 87–89
    shoulder girdle facilitation for lateral weight shifts, 81–82
    sidelying: play in sidelying, 83–86
Prone on Lap, 47–64
    prone lateral weight shifts, 50–52
    prone on lap, 47–49
    prone to sidelying on lap: tactile and visual body
        exploration, 53–55
    prone to sit with extension and rotation, 61–64
    prone to sit with lateral flexion, 56–60
proprioceptive stimulation, 3, 35, 183–184
    over ball, 65–67

    in prone, 47–52
    in sidelying, 53–55
    and transition to sitting, 56–60, 61–64
    in upper extremities, 139–140
pushing, 74–77, 87–89, 106

Q

quadriceps, graded control of, 128–131, 209–214, 226–228
quadruped position, 90, 92
    and climbing, 108–112
    transition from sitting to, 121–123, 124–127
    in transition to standing, 132–133
Quinton, Mary, iii, vii, xiii, xv–xvi, 5–6

R

range of motion, 4, 14–18, 23, 103
reaching, 65–66, 81–82
    active, 11, 24–27, 53–55
    and diagonal weight shift, 152, 162
    to feet, 32–33
    to knees, 19, 20
    and movement from hip joints, 209–214
    and movement to quadruped, 124–125
    preparation for, 70–73
    in prone straddle, 94–95
    in sidelying, 83–86
    in sitting, 139–140
    in standing, 173–177, 220
    and transition from prone, 117–118
    upper-extremity, 11–13, 14–18, 71–72, 161–163, 173–177
    with unweighted arm, 74–77
reciprocal arm swing, 237–239, 240–241
respiration, 80
rib cage and pelvis, abnormal dissociation of, 5
rib cage over stable (fixed) pelvis, 5, 58, 60, 73, 88–89
    and diagonal weight shift, 152–154, 157, 159, 163, 201
    and lateral weight shift, 141–143, 144, 148–150, 192
    in rising to stand, 165–168
    in transition to half-kneeling, 178, 215
righting reactions: in lateral weight shift, 141–143, 144–147
    preparation for, 56–60
    in rolling, 43–44
    in sagittal plane, 185–189
    with sagittal plane weight shift, 203–206
    in sidelying, 39–41, 56–57
rolling: 21–22
    4-month, 34–36, 42
    5-month, 37–41, 43
    6-month, 42–45
    preparation for, 50–52
    symmetrical, 31–33, 38
rotation: around body axis, 61–64, 78–80, 87–89, 97–99
    with extension, 157–160, 161–163, 193–199, 215–218
    with flexion, 152–156, 200–202
    to half-kneeling, 178–181
    to step stance, 219–222
    to unilateral stance, 165–168, 169–172
runner's stretch position, 90–93

and weight shift, 43
visual system, 2, 3, 35
  feedback from, 24–27
  impairments in, 19
  and lateral righting, 74–77, 141–143
  and prone position, 47–49
  and tracking, 11–13, 19–23
  and transition to sitting, 61–64
  and weight shift, 70–73

W, X, Y, Z

walking: cruising and, 234–236
  facilitated from hips, 242–244
  preparation for, 65–67, 165–168, 169–172, 173–177, 198–199, 213, 220–221
  and sagittal plane control, 237–239.
  See also: ambulation
weight bearing: in bear standing, 113–115
  and climbing, 108–109
  preparation for, 128–129
  unilateral, 117–118.
  See also: extended-arm weight bearing, lower-extremity weight bearing, upper-extremity weight bearing.
weight shifts: and climbing, 109
  face-side, 219–222
  to lateral borders of feet, 5, 224–225, 232–236, 242
  onto legs, 128–130, 132–138
  and past-present-future order, 6
  in prone, 83–86
  to reach and play, 81–82
  in rotation to half-kneeling, 178–181
  in sidelying, 56–57, 100–103
  in standing, 173–177
  to symmetrical sitting, 79–80
  and transition from prone, 117–120.
  See also: anterior weight shift, lateral weight shift, posterior weight shift
wheelbarrow, 66
wrist extension, 139–140

Muscles

abdominal muscles: activation of, 19, 23, 92, 226–228
  concentric activation of, 226
  over bolster, 104–107
  in prone straddle, 94–95
  in sidelying, 39, 102–103
  in transition to standing, 134–135
  in walking, 237–239
anterior tibialis, 226–228
dorsiflexors, 129–131, 132–133, 178–181, 226–228
elbow extensors, 139–140
elbow flexors and forearm pronators, 14–18
eye muscles, 11–13, 19–23
finger flexors, 94–95, 97–99
foot musculature, 229–231, 232–233, 234–236
gastrocnemius/soleus muscles, 119, 167, 173–177, 219–222
  in climbing, 113–115
  in rising to stand, 169–172, 209–213
  in transition to sitting, 226–228
gluteus maximus, 97–98, 122, 132, 210–211, 224–225

eccentric activation of, 226
  and gluteus medius, 229–231, 234–236, 242–244
hamstrings, elongation of, 106, 119, 167
  and climbing, 113–115
  in half-kneeling, 216
  in rising to stand, 169–172, 209–213
  in single-limb stance, 221
  in standing, 175–176
  in transition from prone, 117–120
head flexors, 56, 60
  and extensors, 190–192
head, neck, and trunk flexors, 11–13, 14–18, 19–23, 24–27
hip abductors, 113–115, 213–214, 234–236
  and extensors, 108–112, 113–115
hip adductors, 234–236
  elongation of, 124–127, 157–160, 215–218
  in standing, 165–168, 169–172, 173–177, 219–222
hip and knee extensors, 42–45
  over ball, 65–69
  over bolster, 100–103, 104–107
  in cruising, 234–236
  elongation of hip extensors, 31–33, 132–138, 215–218
  in 5-month position, 128–131
  in floor transitions, 117–120
  in preparation for standing, 65–69
  in prone straddle, 94–95
  in rising to stand, 166–167, 169–172, 173–177
  in rotation to stand, 198
  in runner's stretch, 90–93
hip extensors, 74, 76, 78–80, 87–89
  activation of 47–49, 132
  in ambulation, 237–239, 242–244
  in bear standing, 113–115
  over bolster, 97–99, 100–103, 104–107, 215–218
  and climbing, 113–115
  in cruising, 234–236
  difficulty with, 187, 205
  eccentric control of, 213–214, 226–228
  in 5-month roll, 37–41
  and flexors, 203–206
  in half-kneeling, 178–181, 215–218
  with knee flexion, 132–138
  and lateral weight shift, 50–52
  and one-leg stand, 198–199
  in prone straddle, 94–95
  in rising to stand, 166–167, 170–171, 211, 219–222
  with rotation, 61–64, 194–195
  in runner's stretch, 92
  in standing, 213, 224–225, 232–233
  symmetrical, 97–99
  in transition from prone, 117–120
  with trunk extension, 121–123
hip flexors, 21, 56–60, 74–77, 117–120, 185–187, 203–206
  with abduction and external rotation, 156, 181
  in climbing, 108
  elongation of, 47–49, 178–181, 215–218, 242–244
  in 5-month roll, 37–41
  in lateral weight shifts, 50–52
  prone on lap, 47–49
  in runner's stretch, 90–91